BEFORE

TORI BOWMAN JOHNSON

BEFORE – Pregnancy life woman to woman …
The beauty, the bliss, the bothers.
Copyright © 2023 by Tori Bowman Johnson

Written by Tori Bowman Johnson
www.toribowman.com.au | tori@jandvco.com

Illustrated by Catherine Malady

Cover Art by Jacqui Porter

Printed by Mark Print www.markprint.com.au

Designed by Northwood Green
www.northwoodgreen.com | @northwood_green

ISBN: 978-0-6452631-2-1

BEFORE

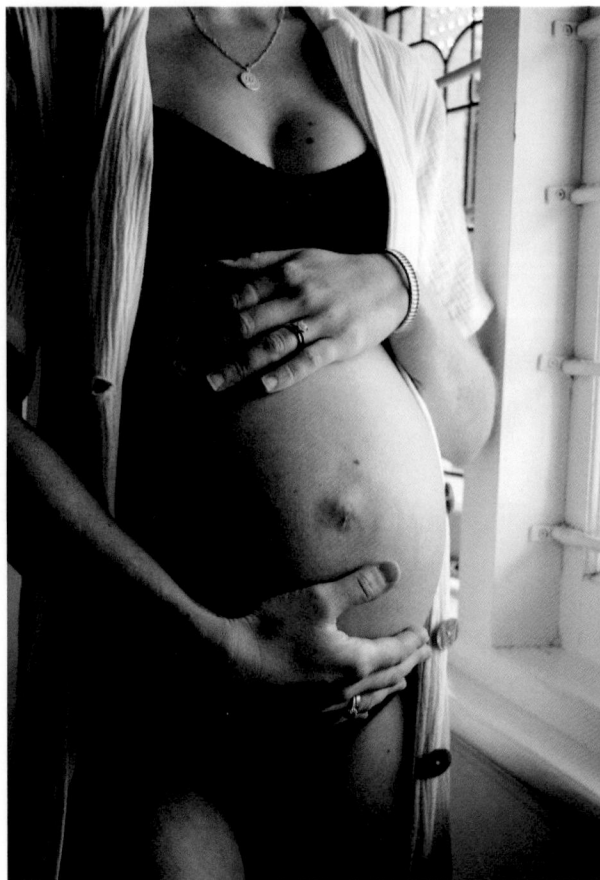

'Well, hold on, darling
This body is yours
This body is yours and mine
Well, hold on, my darling
This mess was yours
Now your mess is mine
Your mess is mine'

– VANCE JOY

To my littlest little, to my George.
Carrying you was carrying the moon.
The sun, the stars, the universe.

Meeting you, was meeting joy.
You have taught me that life is about moving.
Life is about being generous with our smiles
and strong with our bodies.

For giving my Hamish a little brother, I thank you.
For giving me such wholesome purpose,
I cherish you darling.

Whether a baby
is in your belly,
in your arms, in your heart
or tucked somewhere
safely in your future
– you are a mother,
and a sensational
one at that.

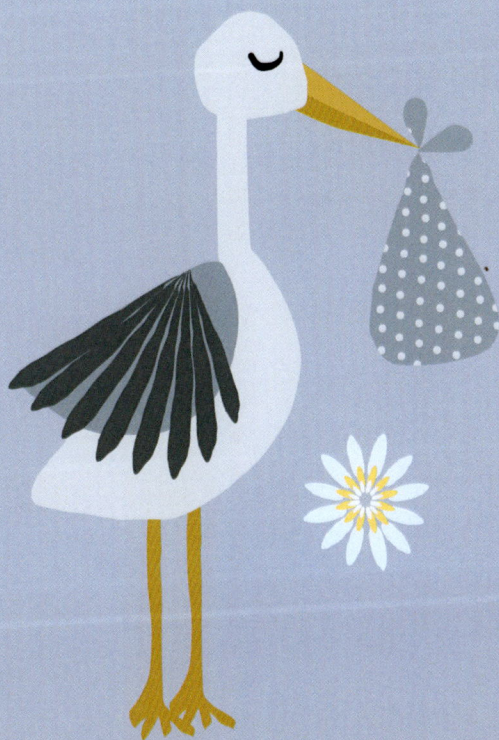

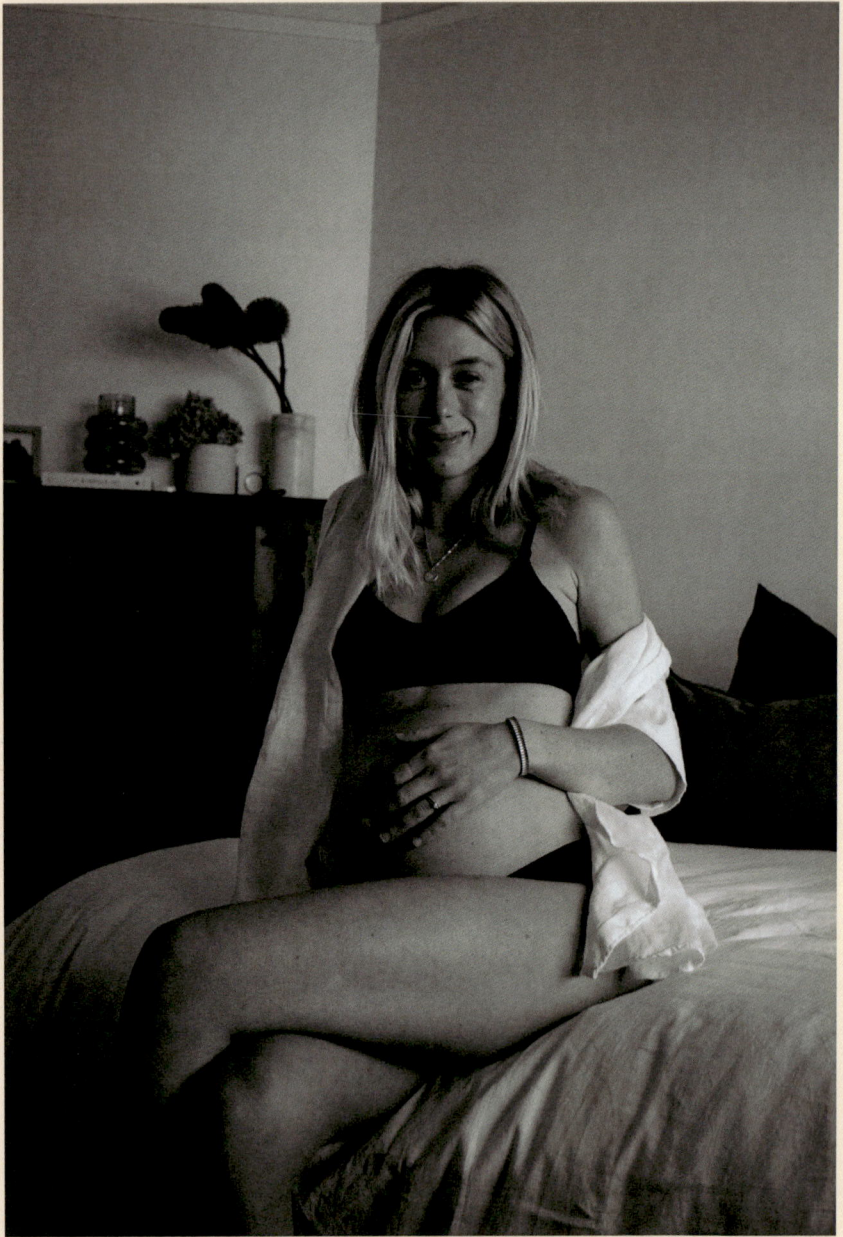

WELCOME

It's me again, hello mummas! This time I'm not writing from the Land of Postpartum but from the Land of Pregnancy. The 9month period of growing a baby! This is now my second baby ... another little body of an unknown soul is sprouting and I feel excited! A second set of arms, legs and organs are expanding inside my very own uterus. How crazy!? But also, how cool! And also... how incredibly bizarre to think that there is a head inside me as well as the one resting on my shoulders!? Ok sorry, that's weird right? Let's move on. Pregnancy, a beautiful time.

The gratitude alone I feel when I'm pregnant is immense to say the least. Especially as this is my second pregnancy and at the age of 32 rather than 29 when I had my number one, Hamish, I'm surrounded by a greater number of friends and family who are commencing their own pathway to motherhood. As my belly grows, as does my, now, toddler Hamish, I can't help but feel tidal waves of guilt at times, as I witness others around me struggling to conceive or experiencing loss and suffering. It just seems too cruel to bare.

The helplessness you feel when you watch others struggle to build a family is dark and dense. It's as if you've just won the lottery and then your best mate loses their job at the very same time. All you wish for, is for everyone who pines for their baby, to have their baby. Right now. In this second. Let them celebrate, like you are.

If you're pregnant too & feeling these feelings just continue to be there for them. Hold back on the advice, the words, the noise. Just listen & be present. I don't really believe there is a parallel to what these women go through. I think their unique experience is something we perhaps shouldn't try to grapple with but rather just let them know they're heard.

For anyone reading who is pregnant (first of all, congratulations!!) and sharing these same feelings of guilt, just remember that while your empathy lends itself wholeheartedly to those around you, let your elation & joy grow too. You can absolutely love & support people while you celebrate something that is special to you. The size of the human heart is immeasurable. Just like the size of your growing belly, your appetite & feed-readying boobs ... *immeasurable.*

I've decided to write this book, the prequel to *AFTERWARDS* if you will, as with each new & pregnant day that passes I'm surprised, alarmed & intrigued by my body. I understand that this is not my first rodeo, however this pregnancy has been wildly different. It's been a lot harder ... so much more exhausting and I am far less interested in what kind of fruit or vegetable my baby is each week, and far more concerned about my exact proximity to Gaviscon & Quick-Eze at all times of the day. If it's location requires me to move further than 6-10 steps to retrieve it, we have an issue.

But WHY is this need so dire?! Why is my indigestion so present this time around but I experienced a grand total of zero last time? Why am I wanting to nestle into a 10 hour nap come 5pm, whereas last time I was energetic & positively buoyant! I actually made my son artwork...using paint ... and a frame! A frame for crying out loud! You couldn't pay me to pick up a pen this time round. I do not feel buoyant. I feel like a bloated blimp.

Pregnancy is remarkable in oodles of way. However to fully appreciate it in all it's glory, I think a greater knowledge of the human body & mind would allow us to be more sympathetic to our needs and more gracious when it comes to our patience. Nothing can be rushed when you're carrying a baby. You have to obey the pace your body assigns you. For some that pace will be indifferent to their usual day-to-day (i.e. me during pregnancy #1) and for others it'll mean applying the brakes on their social lives and purchasing a girdle to hold their tummy up. Ok fine, a 'belly band' or a piece of 'ergonomic supportive wear'... but .... C'mon? Let's call a spade-a-spade hey ladies? Regardless of the fancy name we give it, we're all wearing girdles. It's a vibe.

Like my travels through the winding postpartum roads, there are once again gaps in my knowledge regarding basic human biology knowledge. I have countless curiosities about the many 'taboo' occurrences that happen on the regular over the 9months, and

I am ALWAYS thinking to myself as something new happens to my body, *WTF!?!*

Why do I feel so bloody nauseas from 7am to 7am The Next Day? Isn't morning sickness meant to expire before noon? Why did I get pregnant so easily, but she has yet to experience the same joy after months and months of trying? Why is my hair growing at triple the rate ... while my ability to exercise patience is halving with each week that passes? Why is my sex drive the opposite of what it usually is? All of a sudden why do I need tomato sauce within arms reach, even when I'm not eating?

Why am I living off a diet of Gaviscon, slugged straight from the bottle with a side of hot chips & two minute noodles please (*beef flavour & hold the vegetable sachet*), green apples that have been refrigerated for at least an hour and white potatoes? Why is the sight of my husband's nostrils moving as he breathes causing me to want to stab my fork into a melon? On that note, why does he insist on sitting next to me on the couch when there is an entire floor to be occupied?!

Why do I feel like my body is on fire? So hot!!! But as soon as the wind blows my nipples freeze and it feels like shards of glass are digging into my chest? Why do I need to up the deodorant game, especially when I shower twice a day? Why does the feeling of my thighs touching when I sleep, feel like torture? I used to love my growing body – but now I just feel frumpy. Why do I tear up over... well anything? And everything?!

Why on earth can't I take Nurofen when my whole body aches, or wear the Vitamin A serum that cost me two months worth of my salary. And WHERE the hell is the nearest bathroom?! I NEED TO PEE!

Why does the general public feel as if they need to remind me to sleep as much as I can now before I forever lose the privilege. I GET IT PEOPLE. BABIE'S DON'T SLEEP.

Growing life evolves my curiosities. It is a wild time. My body unfolds with such an innate confidence, while my mind regards the time as precious, yet so peculiar.

BEFORE is going to travel through a myriad of subjects to allow all other curious pregnant women to expand their knowledge and, hopefully feed their patience, their self-esteem ... & of course their will to get up in the morning and fight the urge to eat 3 packets of butter soaked crumpets before 7am.

Bodily changes, keeping well, thoughts on sex, mental health, translating the pregnancy lingo into concepts that are easier to grasp, the processes that make up pregnancies (i.e. scans, tests and the actual birth), and explanations behind the many 'taboo' and quirky elements!

I've been reading some fabulous books & articles of late, written by women who champion and publish with palpable honesty. The types of writers who make you want to pull the words off the paper & hug them because what they write mirrors your own reality. The types of voices who speak to you the way their minds speak to themselves – candidly, spontaneously, always without invitation and yet so comfortably. And naturally.

Honesty is a diluted concept these days, wouldn't you agree? Social media gives us leeway to create and display a certain perspective that, while maybe true, nearly always neglects the surrounding counterparts that make that perspective 'honest'. We live by comparing ourselves to lives that are not fully formed. They're not really lives … they're accounts. It's time to recalibrate and chat openly! The icky, the sticky – the awks! Let's chat about ALL of it!

BEFORE is going to be as 'palpably honest' as possible. For myself, for you. For your pregnant body.

I hope that every woman who reads *BEFORE* – whether pregnant or not – feels as though they can nestle into the notion that 9 months of pregnancy is untypical for every single one of us. We will all experience a different road to birth but the common tie? We're all experiencing a miracle.

It's a beautiful time, an unforgettable time. A time that can't be defined by words or expressions … but it can and should be experienced and enjoyed in good company.

Thank you for being here, *again*. Enjoy!

Tori x

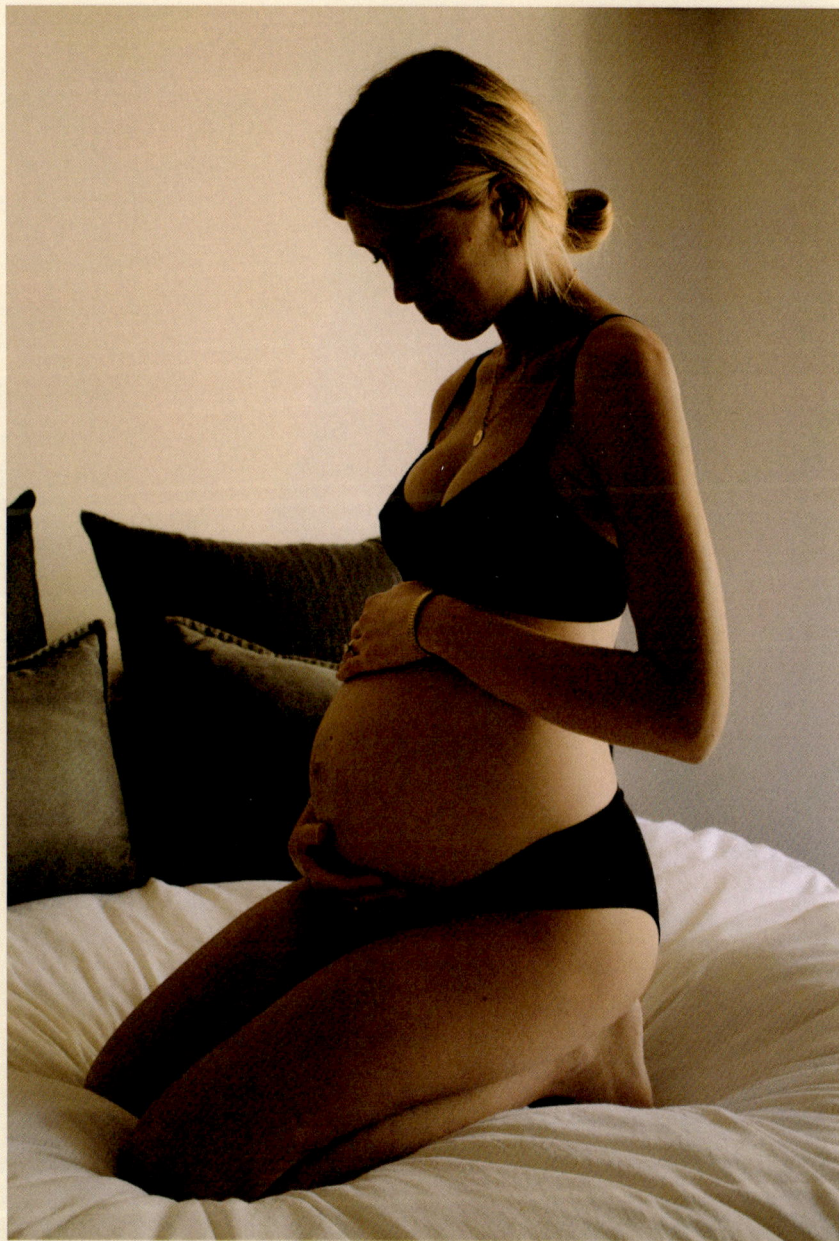

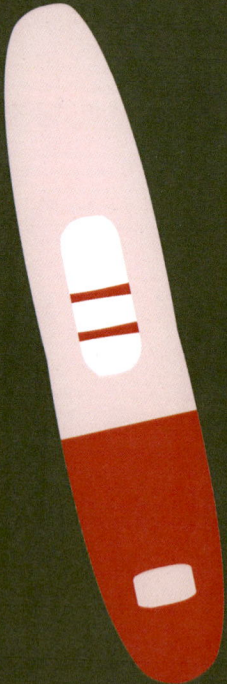

YOU'RE EXPECTING!

MORNING SICKNESS

I feel sick & tired.

Literally. I am writing this particular part of the book
7 weeks pregnant with baby number 2. I had my first scan yesterday and my 1cm
baby bean is happily jumping around with a strong heartbeat. Happy days!

Well yes and no. These 'happy days', aka the First Trimester come with a myriad of
hurdles that can seriously test your will to go on.

Let's talk about Nausea & Fatigue first i.e. morning sickness.

Love this for us prego gals. Ha. Ha.

Firstly let's dissect the term 'morning sickness'. What a load of horse poop this
description is! Morning sickness is actually Permanent, Full Time Sickness for
at least 6-12 weeks for many of us. It feels like a dirty hangover lingering in your
saliva, your stomach, your nasal passage, your whole entire body. Every ounce,
every cell hums with queazy niggles. It is foul.

'Vegemite on toast!!' they say. 'Hydrolytes and ginger tea!!' they say. 'Deep breaths
and midday naps!!' they say. They say a lot, don't they? Everyone means well but
it's exceptionally ballsy to offer a hormonal, nauseated woman advice when she's
on the edge of hurling up her guts. If someone handed me a hot ginger tea during
weeks 6-12, I would have cried a river of furious waves. If I had time for a midday
nap on a day that wasn't a Sunday, I'd fall into a slumber that lasted 8weeks,
leaving my family, my job & my Netflix account to fend for themselves.

What people could & should say that would be slightly easier on the ear is, You
Are Doing So Well. One Day At A Time. I Hear You. I Am Here For. Here Are Some
Hot Chippies ... With Extra Chicken Salt. OR they could give you shoulder massage
while putting their need to breathe on ice. It is universally known that the sound of
a human being breathing makes a pregnant woman's blood boil.

I'm the kinda gal who loves to eat clean. Fresh leafy greens! Rich omegas, fish and grilled chicken and meat. Grains, nuts, fruit in heavy handfuls. Greek yoghurt & long blacks. 'No butter on my toast thank you' & '... dressings on the side please!"

For the last two weeks I've been eating a staple diet of white bread (if I see a grain I'll faint), slathered in yellow butter, bright red jam (I swear the cheaper the brand, the better the taste), or thick, oozing honey. I've been 'snacking' on sausage rolls while replenishing the tomato sauce after each bite, chicken schnitzels, crumpets right out of the bag and I've postponed meetings by 15-30 minutes so I can race down to the local bakery, to order a specific type of pie, pastie or quiche ... or anything else with thick, warm pastry glued to every morsel of fatty meat.

Water is not on my stomach-able list. I've had to dilute my water with lemon cordial just to get it down. HORRENDOUS but ESSENTIAL! Coffee is also a no-go zone 5 out of 7 days a week, so unless I do some exercise in the morning to create energy, I'm reaching for a few red jelly beans to give me a similar morning kickstart. Without it, how would I have the energy to wrangle my toddler, get back to pressing emails or appear on morning Zoom calls with eyes that appear open? My rational mind flatlines at the thought. The jelly beans are crucial.

As I'm reading my words back & proofing, I'm thinking, '...for the love of Pete, 'YUCK. Get a hold of yourself lady!!"

My poor insides! My poor teeth, my poor skin! The poor baby! But this is the reality of early pregnancy right? Those first few weeks or months when you have no control over your stomach. It's a beige shade of grim.

The scary thing is that I'm actually one of the lucky ones. While I'm chowing through all this crap, at least I can keep it down & not have to rely on prescribed medication to control the nausea. The women who depend on anti-nausea meds just to get out of bed everyday, deserve applause. A medal. A cold glass of the world's finest non-alcoholic champagne! Hooray to you superstars. I am in awe of you.

Morning sickness can feel like a never ending, bitch of a hangover. The type of hangover where you're both sick from the 2am tequila shots & completely exhausted thanks to all that sleep you didn't get. It's not a 'pregnancy glow' we adopt is it? It's a hot sweat made up of bacon fat & fatigue.

Let's go back a step shall we? Why do we actually feel this shocking? What is it about a baby growing in our uterus that leads us to feel somewhere on the scale of sea-sick to violently ill & hospitalised?

Well here's the thing. It's not actually 100% known. Crazy right, after ALL this time!? Despite not having an exact cause, the list of 'assumed culprits' include the following:

* Low blood sugar levels
* Changing hormones such as rapid surges in the hcG hormone (aka the human chorionic gonadotropin hormone), and/or changes to estrogen levels
* Fatigue or changing sleep patterns. Having to sleep on your side when you're pregnant is a big adjustment for those who like to sleep on their back or their belly. It can take days or weeks to adjust meaning you may endure some additional feelings of exhaustion.
* Changing diet, including the addition of prenatal vitamins (Hint: Make sure you take your prenatal vitamins at night & after dinner, when your belly is full. If you take them in the morning on an empty tummy or with coffee ... well, good luck to you!)

Around half to two-thirds of pregnant women will suffer from a degree of nausea within their first trimester... and some really unlucky mummas will get the rawest end of the stick. These women – let's call them the Kate Middletons of the world – will be struck down with a condition called Hyperemesis Gravidarum. Hyperemesis Gravidarum is a version of morning sickness so dire it can force women into hospital where they may require a UV drip to rehydrate their system after countless vomiting episodes. Sounds grim doesn't it.

Hyperemesis Gravidarum can actually cause women to lose around 5% of their body weight during pregnancy ... far from ideal! If this situation is resonating with you, please do yourself a favour & seek help. Ask for it, lean into it and then ask for more! The saying 'it takes a village' is true from the moment you decide to conceive.

The fertility journey, pregnancy, birth, postpartum and raising babies ... it ALL requires that village!

So what can help this awful niggling nausea? Let's explore ...

* First of all, don't give it an expiry date based on what friends tell you happened during their pregnancy. Yes, the nausea might dissipate by week 8, 10, 12 or 16... but it also may not. Setting such expectations will only increase the chance of disappointment. Take it day by day. Bucket of hot chips by bucket of hot chips.
* Try to consume Vitamin B when & where you can. For starters, think Vegemite on toast. With Lurpak of course because we are only human.
* If you can stomach it, ginger teas & other herbal teas containing peppermint, lemon or chamomile can help to take the edge off. I found ice-cold tea with lots & lots of ice blocks much easier to digest.
* Taking prenatal vitamins or other supplements such as iron tablets at night and on a full stomach can be much more gentle on the tummy compared to taking them in the morning.
* Snack often during the day to avoid an empty tummy, as this is when nausea tends to feel the worst. Stick to plain snacks such as toast or crackers and avoid greasy, overly sweet, or spicy foods. This can help with heartburn too! Oh & on the topic of heartburn ... if you are suffering with this or indigestion, grab yourself a bag (or twenty) of good ol' Fruit Tingles. Don't overthink this advice ... just hop to and do it! Google it later when you're comfortable.
* Avoid cooking if you can. The smells, the textures, the sights (I'm thinking of you raw chicken), may act as triggers. Pass the cooking duties to someone else, or just stick to your box of crackers.
* Befriend fresh, cool air. Nausea can go hand-in-hand with an increased body temperature, so cooling off outside or under a fan can help. You could even apply a cold compress to your forehead or the back of your neck, which may help to alleviate feelings of nausea.
* Consider your sleeping position. If acid reflux is egging your nausea on or prompting the need to vomit, try sleeping on your left side. Why? The stomach's natural position is on the left. This is where it digests food more easily & effectively. If your vomiting is frequent, try to avoid sleeping on

your back, even in the first trimester when sleeping on your back is still considered safe. **Side Note:** On the topic of sleeping on your back, it is strongly recommended to stop sleeping on your back around 28weeks OR earlier if it helps with peace of mind. According to Pregnancy Birth & Baby Organisation Australia, "Lying on your back puts pressure on major blood vessels. This can reduce the flow of blood to your womb, and restrict your baby's oxygen supply. Research has shown that sleeping on your side can reduce the risk of stillbirth by half." This advice is consistent whether we are talking about sleeping overnight, doing a yoga class, having a facial or simply enjoying a 15minute kip on the couch. Always seek advice if you are ever unsure about safe sleeping positions & never feel too shy to correct someone if they don't accommodate your pregnancy. For example, if you're getting an eyebrow wax, simply ask the therapist to elevate the bed for you. Your body, your call!

* Look into breathing techniques! Deep, slow & controlled breathing can help! Before you roll your eyes & skip this point thinking 'yeh yeh yeh, slow breathing, blah blah blah' just TRY IT! I never embraced breath work before my first birth. Let me assure you, the way you breathe can make a huge difference to the way you feel.

For a starter, try something as simple as breathing in slowly through your nose, hold the breath for 3 seconds & then very slowly breathe out. Repeat this pattern until you feel your nausea start to subside. Why does this work? Nausea can feel like it's something out of our physical control. Breathing techniques are a form of meditation that can recover the sense of control we have over our mind & body, helping us to cope with the physical side effects of nausea.

* Choose to wear looser clothing that won't hug your belly too tight. Whack on a moo-moo if need be! Comfort is key!

* Look into acupressure if you're open to it. Pressing into your bodies acupoints can help muscles relax and improve blood flow.

* Look into acupuncture if you're open to it. Acupuncture (the process of inserting very thin needles into specific & strategic points of your body), can work by stimulating the release of hormones such an endorphins which can block signals to the vomiting centre in the brain & hence reduce nausea.

Hopefully a few of the above ideas above will provide an aid to your nausea. If not, hold on tight & keep hydrated. It won't be forever, I promise.

Oh one last tip on avoiding nausea as we move on ... control what you're forced to smell! Let's dig deeper into this shall we!

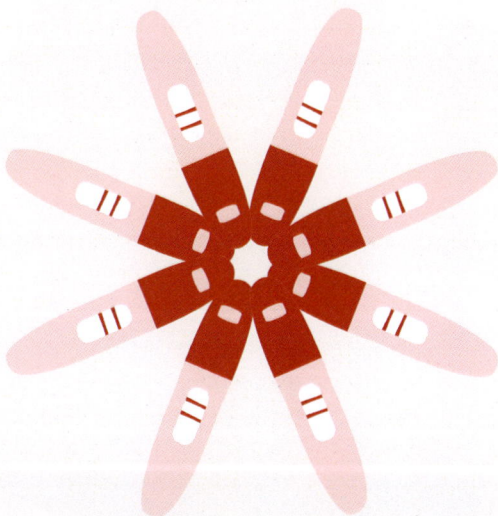

SENSE OF SMELL

This might happen super early in your pregnancy or a little later towards the end of Trimester One, but good gracious me. When your sense of smell changes, it can heighten to the MAX. If someone farted in Florida, I'd smell it.

My deodorant (the original Dove stick with the blue lid), could have been called Wet Dog Smell. Yuck, yuck, yuck! The smell of morning coffee mirrored the smell of canned tuna and don't even get me started with the stench of cheese, artificially scented candles or men who applied aftershave as if they were trying to mask the smell of yesterday's pub crawl ... which ended with a lamb kebab at midnight. The world stank for a good 3 weeks.

This heightened sense of smell is referred to by the medical world as hyperosmia. Like most other things during pregnancy, it's caused by hormones and can be linked to morning sickness in some cases. Understandable, as you don't have to be pregnant to feel crook after smelling something foul.

Unless you're prepared to walk around with a peg pinched to your nose, a few ideas to help you cope with the many offensive smells that crawl up your nose & latch on like stage five clingers, include ...

* Open some windows. Fresh air is the Prince Charming to your nasal passage. Let that bad boy flush your sinuses!
* Refine your use of scented household & wellbeing items.. Fragrance Free dishwashing liquids, soaps and deodorants do exist.
* Look to scents such as lemon, ginger or peppermint when you're feeling off. Cut a lemon in half and give it a good sniff. Sip on peppermint or ginger tea or brush your teeth. Fresh, fresh, fresh.
* Make sure the people around you at work & at home appreciate how sensitive to smell you are right now. If they must eat, cook or clean around you – you need to be warned.
* Bake something that smells yum!
* As for the women who like myself have a toddler and therefore toddler nappies to endure ... my sincere commiserations. Pray.

Smell is one thing to tackle feelings are another. And one common feeling felt by so many women during pregnancy is the feeling of 'I'm fat & frumpy.' Don't beat yourself up if you suffer from this thought. We are all human!

WHEN YOU'RE NEWLY PREGNANT (YAY!) BUT YOU JUST FEEL FAT.

First of all, you're not.

'That Muffin Top' thought. You know that one? Around week 7-10ish ... who else can spot a muffin top make itself a little too comfortable just above their waistline? Me too.

I'm referring to the point during pregnancy when your belly hasn't yet popped but your body has commenced it's expansion journey. Everything looks & feels 'thicker'. Doesn't it?

Well guess what? You are TOTALLY allowed to feel uncomfortable about this change to your body. As women, we are proud beings who have certain expectations in terms of how they'd like to look and feel. When this changes, for whatever reason, it can take some time to adjust. Feeling a little flat as you watch your body change shape and size, does not make you ungrateful or vein. Again, it simply proves you're human.

To make you feel better, here's a personal moment of vulnerability & truth for you. I felt fat and pretty gross for 14 weeks. I was over the moon to be pregnant, for sure! But I was tired, craving crap food, unable to stomach (even look at) greens and I just felt like a tub of lard. Do I feel guilty for admitting to this? To be honest, yes I do. But is it the truth, again yes it is!

Does it define me as a vein, immature woman? God no. I can assure you I am not. I'm reading Diane Keaton's memoir at the moment & I felt slightly better when

I read about the insecurity surrounding her hair. For such a beautiful, iconic & hugely successful woman – even Diane Keaton panders to a crippling insecurity about her appearance, by going to great lengths to buy special shampoo while filling her wardrobe with hats! We are all just learning how to surrender (for like of a better term), to the fact that for a period of time we have to say goodbye to the body we know to be ours. And on top of this we also have to part ways with something so many of us depend on, control.

For as long as I can remember I've always kept fit & eaten a clean diet. During the first trimester of my second pregnancy however, where salad used to sit on my plate, there was now white bread. Basil & lemon seasoning was replaced by tomato sauce from a plastic bottle. A snack went from an apple to a pie. A 3pm 'pick me up' went from a handful of almonds to a bag of lollies.

On two occasions (around weeks7 and 9), I actually took myself to the chemist to weigh myself. Irrational? Well yes considering I had a growing human inside of me … and subconsciously I knew I would only get bigger as the weeks went on, but again, I'm only human right?

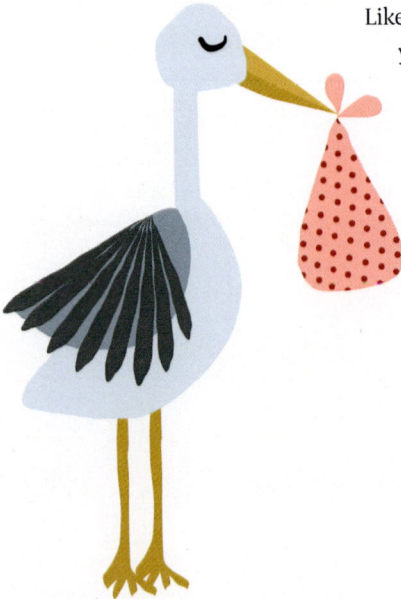

Like postpartum, pregnancy is all about trusting your body & allowing it to take the lead. Don't fret about odd little idiosyncrasics along the way. Just keep on keeping on the best you can. If you need to, pull the car over & grab a sausage roll. Do it.

A Letter to Her Pregnant Self

FROM MILLIE

This mother, Millie, shares a darling child with her wife Jessi. Millie's pregnancy journey included IVF as well as pre & postnatal depression ... yet despite these hurdles, the outcome was their little bundle of sunshine.

Now such a proud mum & hugely celebrated within the LGBT+ community & beyond, Millie writes with power, emotion and such generous love.

Follow their wonderful lives (@jessi_and_millie)

Dear me,

A letter to myself before you were born... 'cause if you had seen this
   was coming, would you have prepared for this storm?

Would you still dismiss these feelings and put them down to
   'baby blues'?
Or would you know to act quickly, because there's really no time
   to lose?
Would you be honest with your family, and say you needed help?
Or would you still just shrug your shoulders, "I guess it's the hand that
   I've been dealt?"

Would you understand that loving your child & feeling sad are not
   mutually exclusive?
Would you be able to decipher the normal thoughts from those that
   are intrusive?

Will you be able to untangle those regular worries about breast or
    bottle fed?
With the unbearable and all-consuming fears, those feelings of
    existential dread?

I would tell you to set those boundaries, and to make sure you hold
    them firm.
Those that matter will understand and the rest will just have to learn.
That No is a full sentence, and that "helpful" advice, you can decline.
Because the 4th trimester is sacred and you will never get back this time.

When the only narrative you hear is "self care"... would you know it's not
    enough?
The community care is the answer, you deserve to be valued, heard,
    appreciated, loved.
Will you still smile sweetly & reply, "Good idea!, You're right!, A hot bath
    would be nice!"
Or would you stand your ground and say, "Washing is a f***ing basic
    human right."

I would warn you that your village might crumble to the ground...
That those you thought you needed, unfortunately, might not stick
    around.
But I will tell you that it's a blessing because you will go on to build
    your own...
And that if you're harbouring these feelings, you're honestly not alone

I know that this seems scary and it's not the type of advice you
    might expect...
But 1 in 4 mums feel this way, and yet we just ignore this subject.
So in case you need to hear it ... you are already a truly wonderful mother.
And if you're feeling sad, or scared or angry – you don't just have to suffer.

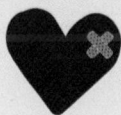

WHERE TO GET HELP

Your GP (doctor)

Maternal and Child Health Line (24 hours) Tel. 13 22 29

PANDA (Perinatal Anxiety & Depression Australia) 1300 726 306

Lifeline Tel. 13 11 14

Beyond Blue Tel. 1300 224 636

Gidget Foundation

Suicide Call Back Service

Professional counsellor e.g. psychologist, psychotherapist

Your maternity or local hospital, many of whom offer support for women (and their families) affected by PND

Maternal and Child Health Nurse in your local council

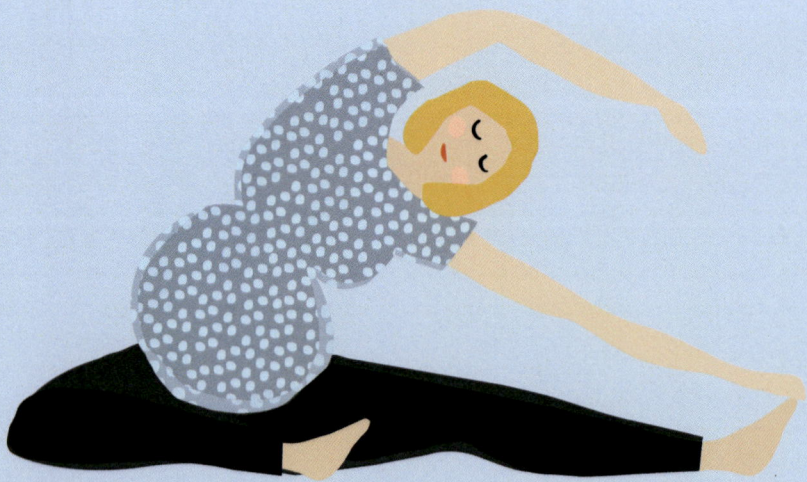

EXERCISE

It's important to note that everything in this chapter is general information only. It is important that when you see the phrase 'Safe During Pregnancy' – whatever is referenced is only considered 'safe' when and if you have personally cleared it with a health professional who knows your body, your pregnancy & your health history in general. Every single pregnant woman is different, as is her pregnancy. There is no 'rule of thumb' and so it's absolutely imperative that you consult your GP/OBGYN/ midwife and/or your women's health physiotherapist before taking on physical activities during your pregnancy – no matter your gestation.

I might sound pedantic and overly cautious, but I am very happy to wear the Pedantic Pam hat if it keeps you safe! Consult & confirm your desired workouts with a health professional before you launch into any physical activity.

And final word of warning before we launch in! Now is not the time to seek a new challenge or chase a PB. If you are not a runner, do not take up running now. If you're not accustomed to weight lifting – do not dive in now! If you don't really do any exercise but you want to move throughout your 9months (good on you!), start with walking (walking in a pool is another option) & perhaps consider introducing guided pilates where you'll have one-on-one support. Ease in!

Ok! Now we have the warnings out of the way – is exercise beneficial during pregnancy? Yes. Some of the major benefits can include reducing the risk of developing postnatal depression, setting your body up for a smoother labour & recovery post birth. There is a chance you may lower your risk of gestational diabetes (I emphasise the word chance here as unfortunately for some women, GD is unavoidable) and pre-eclampsia. Remaining active can also help to lower the risk or the extent of the everyday pregnancy niggles such as constipation, swelling, back aches, pelvic pain & bloating.

In my first book AFTERWARDS (which is all about the postpartum experience as opposed to pregnancy), the wonderfully knowledgeable women's health physiotherapist (and my wonderful friend), Phoebe Marinovich kindly joined forces to guide us through all things pelvic floor. **PELVIC FLOOR.** I am highlighting this because ALL pregnant women need to learn about their **PELVIC FLOOR. Ok? PELVIC FLOOR.**

Phoebe is extremely passionate about women's health when it comes to pregnancy, birth, postpartum, sexual function, continence & general health and education. With a Master's in Physiotherapy specialising in Continence and Gender Health, Phoebe is the specialist we all need in our corner.

This time round, in the pages of BEFORE, Phoebe has come back on board to walk us through exercise during pregnancy, with a particular focus on matters of the **PELVIC FLOOR**.

To put my Pedantic Pam hat on one more time, it needs to be restated that all of the information below is a general guide only. It is not medical advice nor is it a list of instructions to follow. You should always seek guidance & confirmation from a health professional who is familiar with your pregnancy & health history **prior** to launching into any exercise regime. Every woman's body is different, every pregnancy is different & everyones's limitations are different. Vastly different.

Ok, The Basics!

When you fall pregnant, it's a good idea to continue your regular forms of fitness, but to **avoid** taking up anything new. For example if jogging was your jam prior to falling pregnant, you may be safe to continue. In fact, in many cases you might find it's recommended or beneficial! If you're not a runner however – pregnancy is not the right time to start pounding the pavement. Perhaps give brisk walking a go in the meantime or read on for some more ideas.

If you are continuing your usual physical activities, listen to your body in case any niggles or pains pop up. Developing back pain or pelvic pain for example is a sure sign to slow down and seek advice before continuing. Remember that as your body grows & expands, you'll need to make adjustments from week-to-week or month-to-month. A pregnant body requires oodles of TLC.

Below, Phoebe has helped answer a few frequently asked questions on the topic of exercise during pregnancy. This might give you some ideas as to how to safely keep active.

A HANDFUL OF IMPORTANT PRECAUTIONS
(PEDANTIC PAM HERE AGAIN).

A few major notes to keep in mind when embarking on a sweat sesh with your pregnant belly in tow.

1. Keep exercises gentle & moving i.e. in motion. This means that it's good to opt for dynamic rotations instead of elongated holds and sustained stretching. Why? Phoebe explains that you should avoid placing too much pressure on the major blood vessels which affect the flow of blood to the baby. Above all else, keep things comfortable. If it feels painful or uncomfortable – please stop.

   On the topic of stretching, when you're pregnant you may notice that due to the Relaxin hormone produced by your body, you're likely to feel more flexible in areas. While this might feel good, don't let your limber limbs & joints excite you to the point of overstretching. Whether you are pre & postnatal, overdoing the simplest of stretches can lead to discomfort.

   To add more context around the Relaxin hormone during pregnancy, its role is to soften or lengthen , to"relax" the muscles, ligaments and tendons in your joints. The increased flexibility of your hip joints in particular will accommodate your baby passing through the birth canal when it's go time!

2. Exactly when laying on your back becomes unsafe will vary from woman-to-woman and from pregnancy-to-pregnancy. Roughly speaking, between 15-19 weeks is when you should stop laying on your back all together, whether you're exercising or just sleeping. Why? As I mentioned earlier, it's due to the compression of major blood vessels that can compromise blood flow to baby.

3. If you feel breathless or dizzy when standing or laying down during exercise, change position, sit down to rest & hydrate or have something to eat. If the feeling doesn't go away or you lose colour – stop all together & take a seat until you're feeling better. If it continues call your GP, midwife or OBGYN.

4. Abdominal exercises (such as sit ups, bicycles, planks, leg raises etc) are not recommended due to the importance of avoiding tensioning your ab muscles. While we need the tummy muscles to separate and lengthen during pregnancy to accommodate the growing baby, we want to avoid exercises that create too much of a "doming" shape in the midline of the tummy. If you are practising ab exercise, a professional assessment is key to ensure you're not over doing it.

HOW MUCH EXERCISE SHOULD PREGNANT WOMAN AIM FOR?

You should always consult the Australian Guideline from the Australian Department of Health for the most up to date guidelines regarding exercise during pregnancy. A simple Google search will take you to their website (*health.gov.au*).

In short, in many cases engaging in physical activity is better than doing nothing. But ease yourself in! Slow & steady mumma!

To any women who are feeling far to unwell, uncomfortable or simply too busy to exercise – this is OK! Don't let guilt or the frustrating tendency to compare yourself to others inject a sense of failure into your already crowded mind. You're actually doing the opposite of failing, as you're listening to your body & protecting yourself and therefore your baby. Good on you. Rest can be just as important.

HOW WILL I KNOW IF I'M OVERDOING IT?

1. **Exercise the 'Talk Test'** (pardon the pun!) to gauge your limitations while you're getting your sweat on. You should always be able to maintain a conversation while exercising & you should not be able to sing. If you can't talk, this is a clear sign that you are too challenged & you should s low down.

2. **Your body will tell you ...** and you need to listen! Don't try to be a hero mumma – you already are one! Be smart & honest instead.

3. **When in doubt, stop.** No if's or butts!

4. **What "she" can do and is doing, is not what you can do or should do.**
   We are all different! If you are trying to keep up with a friend, or someone you may follow – and you notice that your abilities are not quite mirroring theirs – adjust the workout to suit your body & your needs. There are ways to modify everything.

ABDOMINAL SEPARATION

With talk of pregnancy & exercise, also comes talk of abdominal separation. Heard of it? I'm sure you have! As odd as it sounds to have your abs seperate, it's far more common than you think. To better explain & understand Phoebe has shone some light on the subject, as there is quite a bit to it!

Q. Phoebe, first of all can you please explain what 'abdominal separation' actually is?

PM: Yes! The main muscles concerned with abdominal separation are the "6 pack" muscles (more formally known as the rectus abdominals). Even if you don't think you have a '6 pack' believe it or not, you do! We need this group of muscles to stretch and separate, otherwise how will your tummy expand to allow the baby to grow? Despite not realising every woman's tummy muscles will stretch & seperate during pregnancy thanks to the hormones Relaxin. It's good! We want this to happen.

After birth however, we want these muscles to come back together within the first 3-6months. As everyone has different tissue types & strengths, some women will endure a greater degree of separation compared to others. And in subsequent pregnancies, there is an increased risk of more severe separation.

The aspect of ab separation that most women are probably fearful of is diastasis rectican (rectus diastasis) which is the point where you can actually see the belly bludge, and if left untreated it can lead to poor core stabilisation, pelvic floor dysfunction, and back or pelvic pain.

To avoid a split* to this extent, we recommend that women avoid any exercise that leads to too much doming of the midline where the tummy muscles join. So things like rolling over to get up instead of rolling upwards is a good idea. Avoiding ab exercise such as crunches is also advised. There are still many other ways to exercise your abs during pregnancy so that they maintain strength for birth & recovery. Working with your woman health physio to curate a series of exercises suitable for you & your pregnancy is the best & safest way to go.

In summary, abdominal separation in pregnancy is completely NORMAL. The problem issue occurs however when women are doing too many exercises or day to day movements that worsen the separation.

Q. **If women do experience *diastasis rectican* during their pregnancy, does it lead to a greater chance of having either a C Section or Vaginal birth?**

PM: No. It generally shouldn't affect your mode of delivery.

Q. **Do our abs return to their pre-birth state post birth? If so, how long does it take? How can we help speed up the process?!**

PM: That's the aim for sure & for some this will happen organically. After delivery, within the first 6-12 weeks (or in many cases, within the first year post birth) your body will slowly recover & return to it's "pre-birth state" or a close replica. Realistically speaking, your abs won't necessarily go back to being exactly the same as they were. There may always be a tiny bit of separation & if you go on to have more bubs it's likely the separation will stay or in some cases, worsen. This is very, very common. Women may opt for some guidance using a specific program of exercises to help facilitate the closure of the abs, and a Women's Health Physio is just a phone call away.

Q. **How can we help speed up the process?!**

PM: There is no need to speed anything. Recovery post birth is not a race. Generally speaking however with exercise, postural and breathing advice we can see great improvement in the first 6 weeks or around the 3-6 month mark post delivery.

Q. **What are the symptoms that our abs are splitting too much. Is it true that if we sit up & notice the belly is making a 'triangular shape', it could be a sign of *diastasis rectican*?**

PM: Yes, that is a good test. If you notice that the shape of your belly is significantly "doming" (during pregnancy or postpartum), it's likely that you are working the abs too hard. Like anything, if you are concerned then definitely consult a physio for a professional opinion.

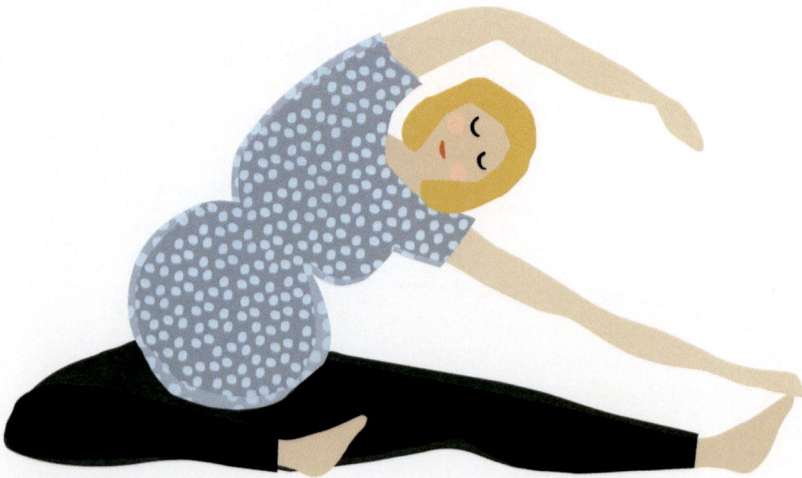

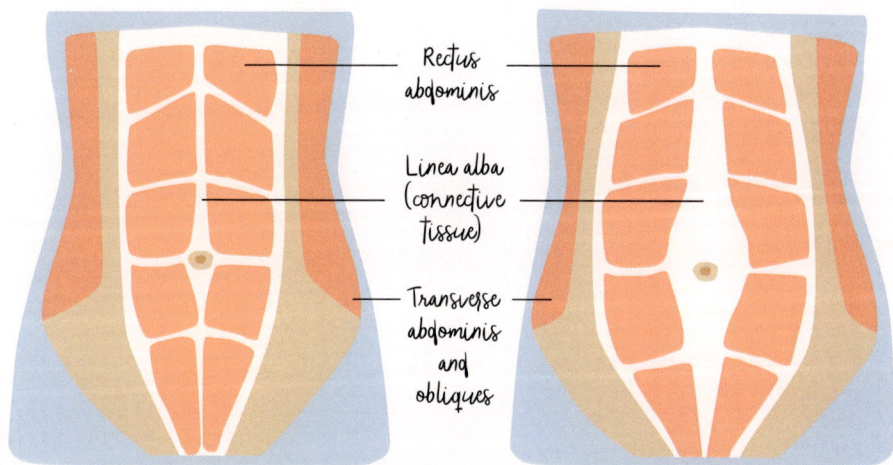

Rectus abdominis

Linea alba (connective tissue)

Transverse abdominis and obliques

Normal abdomen

Diastasis recti

SWEAT SAFE GUIDE

Phoebe has helped me assess a collection of popular exercise styles for pregnancy. Remember that where you see the word SAFE below, it is ONLY considered safe when you have personally consulted a health professional who knows your body, your pregnancy & your general medical history.

SWIMMING

Swimming gets the tick of approval mummas!! The buoyancy of the water will remove all heaviness & pressure from your baby bump and your lower back. You literally feel lighter than your pre-pregnant self in the water, making it such an incredible short-term relief. Swimming can also improve blood circulation & relieve lower limb swelling and discomfort. From someone who swam during pregnancy herself, I swear by it as a fantastic form of daily exercise for both mental & physical goodness.

- ☑ **First Trimester:** Safe
- ☑ **Second Trimester:** Safe
- ☑ **Third Trimester:** Safe, however it's advised to avoid breaststroke kick, particularly for those who are experiencing or who are prone to pelvic pain. Instead, stick to gentle freestyle kick. Using fins & a kick board can be a relaxing option.

RUNNING

Outdoor Jogging & Treadmill
Running can be safe if you're already a runner, but you should always go easy & monitor your breath and heart rate. If you are not a seasoned runner, it's best to take up the hobby after the baby comes & stick to walking or something with less impact for now.

In terms of when to stop running as your 9months progresses, Phoebe advises to let your body be your guide. With this advice, Phoebe also mentioned that most woman will start to feel uncomfortable around 20 weeks (ish), and this is when it's best to slow or stop all together. Remember that you are using a lot of energy to grow your bub, so go easy.

- ☑ **First Trimester:** Safe (if you're already a runner – same goes for Trimester 2&3)
- ⊟ **Second Trimester:** Safe/Proceed with Caution
- ⊟ **Third Trimester:** Proceed with Caution or Avoid if you feel any niggles

Stair/hill running

- ⊟ Again – only if done prior to falling pregnant and your body will tell you when to stop. If something doesn't feel right then stop doing it and modify
- ⊟ From a pelvic floor perspective if you experience any urinary leakage, heaviness etc then stop.

CYCLING

Spin Class

Firstly it's important to refer to the breathlessness scale (i.e. the Talk Test) mentioned earlier in this chapter, to manage your pace & ensure the intensity is modified as you grow. The way you cycle in Trimester 1 will be very different to the way you cycle in Trimester 3 (well it should be anyway!)

- ☑ **First Trimester:** Safe
- ☑ **Second Trimester:** Safe
- ☑ **Third Trimester:** Safe if you go slower!

Road Cycling

Sadly, this style of riding is not recommended unless you're an experienced road cyclist. The added risk of having a fall or being in a road accident is not something you need. And let's not forget pregnancy brain! When you're pregnant it's common to feel distracted & get a little muddled from time-to-time. Being muddled on the road? It's a No from me.

- ☑ **First Trimester:** Safe (if you're an experienced cyclist (same for Trimester 2&3)/ Proceed with Caution

☐ **Second Trimester:** Safe/Proceed with Caution
☒ **Third Trimester:** Avoid

HIIT STYLE TRAINING

Body Weight Exercises
Phoebe has suggested that while HIIT sessions can be OK during the 1st Trimester, during Trimester 2&3 you should proceed with caution and try to consult a qualified trainer who has experience in training pre & postnatal women.

In regards to the core/ab components of each class, you will ALWAYS need to seek advice & guidance before launching into any lower abdominal strengthening exercise. Pretty much everything that engages your stomach muscles (i.e. leg lifts, planks, crunches, toe touches etc) will need to be modified or avoided.

If you're an F45 or HIIT class kinda gal, you can keep going to classes IF you modify as you go and as time passes. When there is jumping involved, you can simply step! When there are weight stations, go light. When there is skipping, grab a latte). Substitute and modify as you go.

I continued F45 classes until I was 37 weeks with my first pregnancy. By the end of it I was pretty much squatting, lunging, doing arm exercises with pilates bands or sitting on the bike for the majority of the 45mins… but just getting to the class & building warmth into my muscles was so good for my body & mind. I was lucky to have a trainer with her eye on me the whole time, which is exactly what every expecting mumma needs.

☑ **First Trimester:** Safe but Modify. Ensure the trainers know you're pregnant (including your gestation if you're comfortable sharing).
☐ **Second Trimester:** Safe but Modify and Proceed with Caution. Ensure the trainers know you're pregnant (including your gestation if you're comfortable sharing).
☐ **Third Trimester:** Safe but Modify and Proceed with Caution. Ensure the trainers know you're pregnant (including your gestation if you're comfortable sharing).

Weight Exercises (i.e. dumbbells)
Heavy weights should always be used with caution or avoided all together for all 3 Trimesters, unless you have a decent amount of experience with weightlifting (or exercise of this nature), and have spoken with your trainer or health professional first. Sorry guys!!

As your body grows, your pelvic floor muscles and pelvic organs are dropping and lengthening. Because of this, adding extra weight will place a heavier demand on the pelvic floor muscles which is unnecessary if avoidable. We need the pelvic floor muscles to maintain their strength for labour & recovery post birth! The less stress you put them under, the fewer pelvic floor issues you'll experience. And in this case, less is more!

Just remember that during pregnancy, the Relaxin hormone loosens our joints and ligaments in preparation for delivery. As a result, high-impact exercises, including weight training, can make you more prone to injury, strains, and sprains.

- ⊟ **First Trimester:** Safe Under Guidance/Heavily Cautioned
- ☒ **Second Trimester:** Heavily Cautioned/Best To Avoid
- ☒ **Third Trimester:** Heavily Cautioned/Best To Avoid

YOGA

It's a big YAY for the yogies! Yoga can be safe during your entire pregnancy BUT always under the guidance of a qualified teacher who should know that you're pregnant. Make sure you listen to your body with each practice, even when you're in a rest or meditative pose such as 'child's pose'. If it doesn't feel right – stop immediately and seek an alternative pose/position.

- ☑ **First Trimester:** Safe
- ☑ **Second Trimester:** Safe
- ☑ **Third Trimester:** Safe

An important note from Phoebe to tack on here regarding Yoga. Hot Yoga should always be avoided during pregnancy. Expectant mothers should not raise their core body temperature above 102 degrees Fahrenheit/38 degrees. Overheating during the first trimester can impact fetal development and can possibly contribute to miscarriage. Later on in pregnancy, it is still highly recommended to put Bikram classes on pause. Any extreme heat may put you at risk of fainting due to low blood pressure and dehydration.

PILATES

Another big YAY as Pilates is considered safe during pregnancy however keep in mind that many exercises during a class will need to be modified. Phoebe recommends that women engage pregnancy specific classes unless they're fully aware & confident in what they can and shouldn't do. Again, like all classes, alert the teacher to the fact you're pregnant.

- ☑ **First Trimester:** Safe
- ☑ **Second Trimester:** Safe
- ☑ **Third Trimester:** Safe

BOXING

Boxing can be safe during pregnancy if it's one-on-one with personal trainer & you can control the amount of pressure & energy you excerpt. It's a good cardio exercise but don't get too fancy with twists & kicks. Keep it simple.

- ☑ **First Trimester:** Safe if one-on-one and controlled
- ☑ **Second Trimester:** Safe if one-on-one and controlled
- ☑ **Third Trimester:** Safe if one-on-one and controlled.

TEAM SPORTS

Not recommended but if you MUST, be careful, be sensible & remember you are pregnant!!! If there are balls, bats, sticks, skis, boards, rackets or kicking involved – think about taking up swimming?! I am the most risk averse person you'll ever meet but when it comes to carrying a baby, I'll never apologise for my conservative side.

If you do play a game of tennis or go for a ski, if there is any contact with your abdomen, please call your OBGYN, midwife or your GP right away. Even if you feel OK, call them anyway and tell them what happened. This advice goes for ALL sports, activities & general daily tasks. At 37 weeks I tripped on a cord and fell forwards onto my knees. The impact was quite shocking but I didn't hit my tummy – so I didn't call my midwife. By coincidence I saw her the next day and got a big tell-off. And rightly so. You can never be too careful.

- ☒ **First Trimester:** Not Recommended/Proceed with Caution
- ☒ **Second Trimester:** Not Recommended/Proceed with Caution
- ☒ **Third Trimester:** Not Recommended/Proceed with Caution

PELVIC FLOOR EXERCISE

The condition of your pelvic floor is very important during pregnancy ... and just in general to be honest. Firstly as we're covering the subject of PF health in the Exercise chapter, the question might dawn on you, 'Do pelvic floor exercises count as 'exercise'?' Phoebe explains, sadly no. They don't count as exercise per se (i.e. cardio or strength) but they should incorporated into your daily routine.

Like that old saying 'It's better to ask for forgiveness rather than permission', this is a similar theory to the matter of your pelvic floor. You're much better off strengthening your pelvic floor BEFORE the arrival of your baby rather than working to recover & strengthen it AFTER the birth – regardless if you deliver vaginally or by c-section.Much, much, MUCH!

I've cut & pasted a direct excerpt from my first book, AFTERWARDS (all about Postpartum) below which covers everything under the pelvic floor banner. Throughout AFTERWARDS, Phoebe helped define & explain what we need to know, so it's all here again to refresh our understanding.

PELVIC FLOOR CONT.

Let's dig deeper into the PF shall we?

Q. Let's Recap. What is the Pelvic Floor?

PM: The pelvic floor consists of muscles & fascia (i.e. connective tissue) located inside the pelvis. The pelvis is a complex of bones that connects your trunk to your legs.

The pelvic floor muscles are a group of muscles that sit like a hammock at the base of your pelvis. They work to keep us continent (in terms of both our bladder and bowel), they support the pelvic organs (i.e. the bladder, bowel & uterus), and they support the lumbar spine with the lower abdominals. Finally, the pelvic floor muscles support sexual function. They are very important in terms of arousal and climax.

THE IMPORTANCE OF THE PELVIC FLOOR

Q. Now let's go over the role of the pelvic floors during pregnancy & after pregnancy? And how it works in relation to the uterus & the vagina.

PM: During pregnancy there is a lot of added pressure and weight on the pelvic floor due to the baby growing inside of the uterus. From the size of a blueberry, they grow into a melon before you know it! Due to the growing weight, the pelvic floor muscles have to work harder than ever to keep us continent, and to support the pelvic organs.

The hormonal effect of pregnancy (particularly the addition of the Relaxin hormone), causes our ligaments, our fascia and our muscles to soften in preparation for the birth. The softening effect also occurs to accommodate the baby in the uterus. With all of this in mind, during pregnancy a woman's pelvic floor needs to perform!

After the baby is born, the pelvic floor muscles are not off the hook just yet. They're required to get back to work asap. Back they go to holding everything

UP and IN. As the pelvic floor has been working over time during the 9 month pregnancy, it's not uncommon for the pelvic floor to be tired and weak. Anyone finding themselves weeing a little when they cough, laugh or sneeze? If so, this is a classic example of the pelvic floor lacking the strength to retain full control.

For this reason, women really need to add some extra TLC into their day to ensure they regain their strength asap post birth. Particularly for women who would like to have more babies. If you can prioritise and nail a full or at least a decent recovery, your body will cope much better when it's time to grow and birth another baby, compared to if you became complacent or lazy after baby #1.

Q. **The best way to regain strength and control of the pelvic floor?**

PM: Exercise!

Gentle exercises post birth can be great when practiced **correctly** and **regularly.** Generally speaking, it should be ok to commence some gentle exercises straight after birth (as long your catheter is out. However before launching in, it's absolutely encouraged to get the official OK from your maternal health nurse, your GP or your women's health physio.

Before we explore some exercises, let's address a very common question;"How long will it take my Pelvic Floor to recover post birth?"

This is the million dollar question & unfortunately one with no definitive answer. Your recovery time will depend on a number of varying factors, including of course your genetics, your pregnancy & your birth.

* Those who endured a traumatic delivery may encounter a decent amount of swelling, bruising or even more severe damage. This can take some time to heal & these women might be a little late returning to the trampoline.
* Those who are genetically blessed & have very elastic, stretchy skin around their downstairs region may bounce back a little sooner.
* Those who are diligent & committed to practising regular pelvic floor exercises & prioritise visits with their women's health physio, may notice an accelerated recovery time as well. Working with a women's health

physio is an incredible way to receive guided feedback regarding your body. It's important to keep reminding you that matters of the pelvic floor are unique to each individual. What you require is not what they require.

* Those who suffered a prolapse post birth or a partial prolapse may encounter a slightly more uphill battle in terms of their recovery as their setback is a little more complex.

This list could go on but it's best not to fuel your mind with worries & override positive thinking. Especially as it's **never** too late to strengthen your pelvic floor. You are not broken. The life & times of your vagina does not have to be defined by your choice to be a mother. But try and surrender to the fact that it takes time, work (and rest), patience & self awareness.

As mentioned, there are so many contributing factors to the recovery of a woman's pelvic floor after birth. As you're on the road to recovery, remember that even though your stitches may have dissolved & your vagina appears to be less swollen, never discount what is going on internally.

Birth doesn't just affect the side we can see. The birth canal, the uterus, the bladder ... all of these internal parts of your body have gone through a hell of a time. They'll be bruised and tender so at the very least, go easy on yourself. Show your body the respect it deserves & in due course it'll return the favour.

Before we move onto exercises, make sure to remind yourselves that pelvic floor health & strength is not only related to pregnancy and birth. It's an area of your body that requires focus & attention at all times, or both females and males.

THE KEGAL EXERCISE

Q. The Kegel, please explain?

PM: The Kegel is an exercise that works the pelvic floor muscles. It's almost like a "vaginal squeeze" and internal lift sensation.

First up; the best way to ensure you're exercising the right area is to make sure nobody can detect you're doing your Kegel s when you're doing them! If your buttocks and thighs are lifting, you're not using the right muscles.

Q. How exactly does one practice the Kegal?

PM: Very simply ... and the best thing is that you can do them wherever & whenever.

* Imagine you are sitting on a small marble ball & you are trying to lift the marble up using your vagina. Another thought, imagine there is a straw in your vagina and you're using it to suck liquids upwards.
* As you feel the upwards squeeze, now imagine as if you're simultaneously trying to hold in wind.
* Identify this feeling as you squeeze, hold & release.
* As well as your buttocks and thighs, nothing higher than your belly button should move or contract while doing your Kegel s. And avoid holding your breath!

Q. How many & how often should we be doing them? Is it the same advice for both pregnancy & postpartum?

PM: Yes and no. Kegels can be executed during both periods, however the amount can be individualised to the person, especially as birth is nearing. For example if you're someone with an overactive PF, then you want to focus on the relax part. This is where you are best off working with a women's health physio to understand the condition of your PF.

To explain how to do your Kegels:

* Hold each Kegel for 3-10 seconds & repeat them 5-10 times.
* In the very early postpartum days when you're still recovering, be very gentle & take it slowly. It's always recommended that you check with your midwife, maternal health nurse or women's health physio before commencing your vaginal workout.
* Aim for a few sets per day. A nice way to remember to do your exercises is to do them while doing another daily task, such as taking a shower. If it becomes associated with an existing routine, you are much less likely to forget. Breastfeeding is another good time to focus on you getting your Kegels in.

If you practice daily Kegels before and during your pregnancy (first of all, good on you!), you may notice that following the birth the exercise might feel quite different & quite possibly more difficult. This is normal. Don't panic!

To explain the difference, the muscles will be fatigued & slightly weaker due to the 9 months of pregnancy and the birth. Do your best to solider on with your Kegels though, as it will assist with the healing process and it might even help to reduce swelling.

WARNING: Practising Kegels while doing a wee (i.e. by trying to stop your wee mid-stream is **not** advised). The "wee test" is not a good habit to fall into as it can create negative bladder habits.

To wrap up the wonderful subject of exercise … Daily movement & gentle exercise during pregnancy is fantastic! Stick to your usual routine & make modifications as you go (week-to-week or even day-to-day if need be!). EVERYTHING should be checked with your health professional BEFORE launching in & if you're in a group class or under the guidance of an instructor, it is recommended to tell them you're pregnant so they can monitor you carefully. Health and safety is everything when a baby is on board.

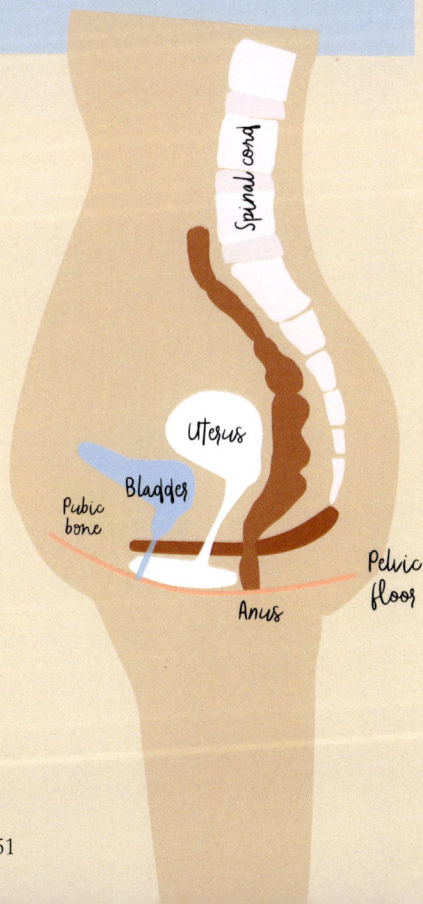

Spinal cord

Uterus

Bladder

Pubic bone

Anus

Pelvic floor

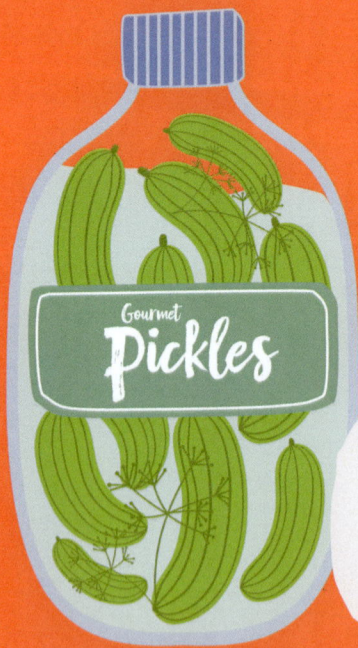

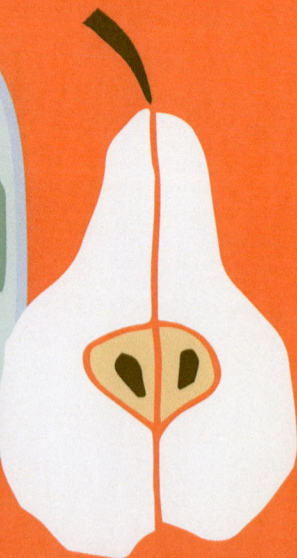

FOOD & NUTRITION

Food. Oh how we love it! Yet how we seem to have such a complicated relationship with it throughout pregnancy, especially during the infamous 1st trimester. Some women will have an aversion to absolutely everything, some women will have an aversion to almost everything unless it's white, cooked in spitting fat and covered in three kinds of salt – table, Himalayan & chicken. Others will remain unfazed & hungry for what they're usually hungry for.

While cravings & aversions can change by the second – the major goal throughout the 9months is to try your best to consistently devour as much nutrients as possible. For both your own health & the health of your growing baby.

Luckily for us, we have a wonderful OT and Nutritionist with a keen interest in maternal and bub health, Caroline Harangozo, with us for this chapter to walk us through the many aspects of eating and nutrition whilst pregnant. You can find more of Caro's inspiring recipes at @caroline.otnut.

A mother herself to handsome little Banjo, Caro has filled this chapter with palatable advice & insightful information to help us understand how & why food can have such a profound effect during pregnancy. If you can understand 'the why' in particular, then like anything, you'll find it easier to adopt & action.

Caro has also squashed a few old wives tales & shone a light on various considered advice. From dealing with unusual cravings, to being diagnosed with Gestational Diabetes, to lending her knowledge to the food options we can focus on to make sure we get adequate protein, folate, iron & other important vitamins and minerals.

Welcoming Caro into the book is beneficial for us all!

Let's talk foods that can help combat sugar/salt cravings in Trimester One? Please enlighten us Caro!

CH: First of all people should know that pregnancy cravings are very normal and very common during the 1st & 2nd trimester in particular. And with cravings, can also come food aversions.

It's still not known why pregnancy causes certain cravings, however as you can imagine, there are many theories. Some believe we crave the dietary elements we are nutritionally deficient in. For example, craving red meat might be your body's way of telling you that you are deficient in iron. While it makes a level of sense, there is limited scientific evidence to confirm this theory is entirely true.

Pregnancy aside, cravings for most point to an imbalance in blood sugar levels. If we prioritise eating balanced meals (including snacks) throughout the day, then we are less likely to have radical cravings for super sweet or salty foods.

On the topic of salt, it's helpful to know that our bodies need for salt increases in pregnancy, due to the greater amount of fluid in our body. In turn this increases the need for electrolytes, and therefore we require more minerals in our diet such as salt. Sprinkling some salt to season our foods is a good way to tackle this.

We often snack more when we are pregnant and snacking on balanced snacks is a good way of helping to control our blood sugar levels throughout the day. Like meals we want our snacks to ideally contain carbohydrates, protein and fat to stop our blood sugar from spiking. Some examples of 'balanced snacks' include a piece of fruit with a side of nuts or nut butter, pairing savoury crackers with a slice of cheese and tomato, having a slice of wholemeal or multigrain toast with avocado, hummus or a boiled egg and whole fat plain yoghurt with fresh berries and \nuts & seeds.

During the 1st trimester, the nausea some women endure can be so intense that eating balanced meals becomes difficult. The priority here is to eat something rather than nothing and do whatever you can to keep hydrated. If you suffer from severe nausea during pregnancy and it's affecting your ability to stomach most foods I would encourage you to work with a nutritionist or a dietician during this time so you can be provided with individualised advice or at least consult your GP. A final note that I think is valuable – a balanced diet is one that contains enough carbohydrate, fat & protein (and calories) so we're left feeling full and nourished. If we are satisfied and our blood sugar levels are controlled, we're much less likely to reach for the cookie jar or hot chips between meals.

Q. **Now, how about foods we can eat to help us avoid Gestational Diabetes?**

CH: Gestational Diabetes is not always avoidable unfortunately. For some, it's out of our control but for others there are a few ways we can decrease our risk. A whole-food diet for starters, that is high in good quality proteins, fibre, meets nutrient requirements and that is low in sugar & processed high glycaemic carbohydrates is encouraged. Ideally we want to try and minimise foods like processed cereals, cakes biscuits, pastries, fruit juice, soft drinks etc. where possible. Carbohydrates are not inherently unhealthy – however when we eat them we should aim for less processed and wholegrain carbs and pair them with good quality fats and proteins to stabilise blood sugars.

On top of diet, exercising regularly throughout pregnancy can help to lower your risk of Gestational Diabetes. The risk factor can be decreased by up to 70%! Before falling pregnant, working on getting to a healthy weight is advised. Carrying excess kilos prior to conception is a 'modifiable risk' factor for Gestational Diabetes. If you're planning to have a baby, making some healthy lifestyle changes is important.

Genetics also plays a role. Having a family history of Gestational Diabetes is a 'non-modifiable risk' factor of developing GD, and although diet and lifestyle is still optimum, for some there is simply no way to avoid the diagnosis. Instead the focus needs to shift from avoiding GD to effectively managing it – which is possible!

Q. **For those who are unlucky and are diagnosed with GD, what are some food examples to help manage it?**

CH: If you are diagnosed with GD, firstly know that you are not alone. Gestational Diabetes is the one of the most common pregnancy complications and affects approximately 15-20% of pregnant women.

Limit sugar intake and processed foods and focus on meals with high quality protein and fat sources, lots of non-starchy vegetables and moderate amounts of wholegrain or unprocessed carbohydrates.

The key is to consume foods that sustain your appetite and will thus regulate your blood sugars. Regularly test blood sugars after each meal and learn what foods/meals increase your blood sugar and which ones do not.

Nutrition & exercise should be the primary treatment to help manage GD but when this is not sufficient, women may be prescribed insulin or other medication.

If you do have GD, you'll need to be under the care of a multidisciplinary team whose job it is to help you manage your blood sugar levels. It's imperative you obtain individualised advice as GD is not a 'one size fits all', and inadequate management can cause problems for your baby and you (e.g. it can cause babies to be born larger, be born hypoglycemic, increase the risk of lung problems and shoulder dystocia and it can also increase the risk of baby developing diabetes when they're older). There is also a higher chance of birth intervention such as a C-Section.

Side Note: For those who do have a diagnosis of Gestational Diabetes or it runs in your family & you're trying to conceive, I would highly recommend getting yourself a copy of the book, "Real Food in Gestational Diabetes" by Lily Nichols. She's an expert when it comes to GD and nutrition.

Q. **We spoke about cravings earlier, so how about we move onto the topic of the dreaded nausea. When nausea hits, how do we manage?!**

CH: Nausea during pregnancy is tough – really tough!! Hang in there & cross your fingers that in your case it may subside during the later stages of the 1st trimester.

Working out, early on, exactly what your nausea triggers are can be beneficial to help stop them in their tracks. It might be certain smells, sights or textures. Your sensitivities may be worse at particular times of the day i.e. easing your nausea could be as simple as making sure you eat something as soon as you wake up in the morning. Make notes when you're having a tough moment & see if you can identity a pattern.

I've listed a few tips below:

* Eating smaller meals more frequently throughout the day will mean you don't get too hungry or too full. This will help prevent your blood sugar dropping which can make nausea worse.
* Look to foods that are easier for your stomach to digest. Smoothies and soups are a great example of this. You can make them nutrient dense and, depending on the ingredients, they are easier to stomach.
* Carbohydrates are the easiest types of food to digest when we're feeling nauseous, so focus on good quality carbs when you can. Think potatoes with their skin on, wholegrain bread and crackers and brown rice.
* It's not uncommon to wake up feeling nauseous first thing, so having snacks by the bed can help. Think plain or wholegrain crackers, nuts or a banana.
* Take your time to eat, eat mindfully and chew your food. Get rid of the phone or the laptop … sit & enjoy your meal.
* Ask someone else to prepare your meals (a parent, sibling, friend or your partner) or have meals pre-prepared in the freezer. These ideas require a support network & a level of organisation but they can be a mega help if you lean into either.
* Try to avoid drinking too much liquid at mealtimes.
* Steer clear of high fat meals & snacks as they are much harder for the stomach to digest.
* Load up on ginger supplements, ginger tea or dried ginger. Ginger has anti-inflammatory properties & and it can improve digestion. On top of this, the spice supports the release of blood-pressure-regulating hormones which relaxes your body and reduces feelings of nausea.
* Sometimes B6 supplements can help with nausea or consuming foods high in B6. Examples include potatoes and sweet potatoes, bananas, avocados and pistachios. Meats and fish are also high in B6 however understandably these can be hard to stomach. But if you can, eat up!
* Seek help from your doctor if you are not coping with nausea. There is medication that can help with severe nausea and it helps to get on top of the nausea early, rather than waiting until you can no longer eat or drink anything or keep anything down.

Q. When the nausea is dire & even water brings on the ick-factor, what are the most important types of food you should *try* and eat?

CH: If you can't keep anything down, you will most likely need to focus on bland foods that your stomach can digest without too many issues. This will differ from person to person but generally speaking, things like plain toast, salty crackers, carbonated drinks (for example ginger-ale or lemonade), broths and/or flavoured water (Hydralytes are good for this). If you can't keep anything down you must contact your doctor as dehydration, especially when pregnant, can be very dangerous.

If you're vomiting, you'll need to replenish lost fluids and electrolytes quickly. Sip on electrolyte drinks (again, Hydralytes are good for this), icy poles, cold coconut water, smoothies, broths or fruit juices that have been diluted with water. And consuming salty foods is another option.

During these very rough days/weeks – don't worry too much about maintaining a balanced diet. For most people our bodies are smart, intuitive and they'll have enough nutrient stored to look after you and the bub during this time.

Eating something is better than eating nothing, so if potato chips and lemonade are the only thing you can stomach for a short period of time, then so be it!

When pregnant, we are commonly advised to take supplements containing ingredients such as folic acid, iron and calcium. As well as maintaining general wellness with diets high in protein, omegas & fibre – these three particular vitamins & minerals are exceptionally beneficial during pregnancy.

Before leaning into Caro's knowledge, firstly let's just break down What & Why we need folic acid, iron and calcium in particular as when you're pregnant these are words you will hear a lot!

FOLATE

Folate falls within the Vitamin B family and it's role is to support healthy foetal development. During the early days of pregnancy, folate helps to form your baby's nervous system and neural tube. Inadequate folate can increase the risk of neural tube defects such as spina bifida, so taking it is advised. While it can be efficient to introduce a pregnancy safe supplement into your diet, we can also find folate in food & therefore work it into our daily diet. Keep reading for further details.

IRON

When you're carrying a bub, the volume of blood in your body increases, as does the amount of required iron (hence why many women take iron supplements at some point over the 9 months). Your body uses iron to make more blood so that during the pregnancy it can supply enough oxygen to the baby via the placenta.

Iron is also very important for bub's development, so it's important to measure your iron status during pregnancy. Low iron (signs of which may include feelings of lethargy, lightheadedness & an inability to concentrate), can increase the likelihood of a premature baby, the bub having a lower birthweight and neurodevelopmental delays. Low iron levels can also increase your risk of infection – so it's VERY wise to keep on top of your iron levels via regular blood tests. Your OBGYN, midwife or GP should be all over this.

Hot Tip: If you do end up taking iron supplements, consider upping your fibre intake as iron supplements are famous for causing constipation. You may also need to take something to help with the constipation if it becomes prolonged or uncomfortable. Chat to your GP if this happens as you can also swap the type of iron supplement you are taking which might also help.

If constipation leads to excess straining on the toilet, this can lead to Haemorrhoids – and nobody likes those! To get ahead of this cycle, say hello to added daily fibre, drink lots of water and remember to move throughout the day.

CALCIUM

Your growing baby needs calcium to form strong bones & teeth. Think about it this way, your baby has an entire skeleton to build from scratch! Adding to this, calcium is an important nutrient for your baby's heart, muscles, nerves, and hormones. Calcium can also reduce the risk of hypertension and pre-eclampsia.

Q. Moving on to foods with these vitamins & minerals. Let's start with folate! What types of foods are rich in folate?

CH: You can find folate in foods such as nuts, seeds, avocados, eggs, beans, peas, lentils and green leafy vegetables (think broccoli, spinach & kale).
Folic acid is the synthetic version of folate and is found in some prenatal supplements. Not everyone is able to metabolise this synthetic version of folate so I recommend you get suitable guidance by a health professional trained in this field when choosing the right prenatal supplement or folate supplement for yourself.

Q. Which types of foods are rich in iron?

CH: As mentioned earlier our iron needs are much higher during pregnancy (about 1.5 times higher), so we need to load up.

You can find rich sources of iron in:

* **Heme-iron foods** (i.e. foods derived from animals) as they are absorbed more efficiently compared to non-heme foods (i.e. plant-based iron). Foods rich in heme-iron include salmon, sardines, lamb, chicken, beef, turkey, bone marrow and duck/chicken liver.
* **Foods rich in non-heme iron** (these foods include dark green leafy vegetables, broccoli, seeds, nuts, quinoa, black beans, kidney beans, lentils, chickpeas, seaweed, tofu, tempeh, potatoes with skin on, prunes, olives, apricots, dark chocolate too!) it's > 50%.

HOT TIP! Foods containing iron should always be consumed with foods that are high in vitamin C. This will boost iron absorption.

Q. Which types of foods are rich in protein?

CH: Ok, protein! An important part of your pregnancy diet! Similar to iron, our protein needs increase during pregnancy. They actually continually increase as the pregnancy progresses. For example someone at 30 weeks will likely need more protein than someone at 16 weeks.

Consuming an adequate amount of protein is required for optimum foetal development. Protein rich foods will also help stabilise blood sugars and keep us full. Adequate protein consumption can also help with fatigue, food cravings (especially in terms of sugar!) and nausea as it helps to control our blood sugars.

Foods rich in protein include:

* Red meat (grass fed)
* Fish and other seafood
* Poultry (pasture raised)
* Eggs (make sure they're cooked through; avoid runny eggs).
* Bone broth and collagen
* Dairy products (cheese and full fat yoghurt)
* Nuts and seeds
* Legumes

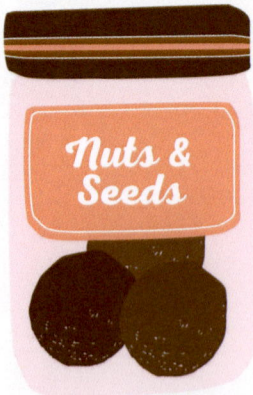

Q. Foods that are rich in omegas?

CH: During pregnancy it's also essential to consume the omega 3 fatty acid DHA via diet or supplementation. pregnancy. Note, food consumption is preferred over supplementation where possible.

DHA is needed for brain & eye development. It also protects the brain from damage and inflammation.

The best food sources of DHA include fatty fish such as salmon, sardines, tuna, herring and trout. You should aim for 2-3 serves a week.

There are also good levels of DHA (albeit less than fatty fish) in chicken, eggs (pasture raised) and beef (grass fed). After seeking medical advice from someone such as their OBGYN, midwife or GP, vegans and vegetarians may also consider high quality DHA algae supplements to ensure they are meeting their DHA requirements.

Q. Moving on, what foods should we think about eating AND avoiding when and if we suffer from heartburn or indigestion?

CH: Heartburn is another very common pregnancy complaint! Over half of all pregnant woman have it at some point during their pregnancy. This is due to increased pressure on your stomach due to the growing baby, increased acid in your stomach due to the placenta producing gastrin (gastrin acts to increase levels of hydrochloric acid in our stomach), slower intestinal movement, and increased progesterone levels which relaxes the oesophagus sphincter.

Things you can do to manage heartburn or indigestion include:

* Eating small meals and snacks rather than large portions.
* Sip on liquids throughout the day rather than consuming a lot of liquid at meal times.
* Some people swear by drinking a small glass of water with some added apple cider vinegar (a teaspoon or so) before eating to help with digestion.
* As heartburn is often worse at night when we lie down, try to eat smaller

dinners at an earlier time. The earlier time means you'll be walking around before bed which will help to settle your stomach.

* Often caffeine, spicy, high sugar or acidic foods, and foods containing dairy or gluten can make heartburn worse for some people. Try excluding some of these foods and see if it helps – keeping a food diary can help.

* Good posture helps as there is more room for your stomach to do its job of effectively digesting food, so try to sit tall when eating and after eating.

* For both heartburn & indigestion – people swear by Fruit Tingles. (Note from Tori on this point … Fruit Tingles SAVED ME! A few after meals is all that it took to prevent a night of horrible indigestion. I actually found them to be more effective than QuickEze and Gaviscon). Fruit Tingles contain sodium bicarbonate which is thought to be the magic ingredient. If you have toddlers, make sure they're kept well out of reach as they can be a chocking hazard.

Q. Ok. I have to know. Eating for two (or more if you're carrying multiples!). Is this true?!

CH: Not really, I'm sorry to say!

Our calorie needs do increase slightly but not enough to feed two people. Our calorie needs will also depend on how much physical activity we are doing and what stage we are in our pregnancy. They'll increase the further we progress as our bodies use more energy to grow the bub.

Something to be mindful of is that some women will need to monitor their calorie intake based on the amount of physical activity they engage in. If they're less active, their calorie intake may not need to increase at all. Roughly speaking, our calorie intake increases enough to add 1-2 extra snacks per day. You may find that some days you feel hungrier than others – so it's important to eat mindfully and tune into your hunger cues.

Although our calorie needs doesn't increase too much, what **does** increase is our need for particular micronutrients such as B12, iron, iodine, folate, choline, calcium and omega 3s.When we are pregnant, we should focus on eating a nutrient dense & wholefood diet rather than just eating larger portions. Quality over quantity!

Q. Dehydration can be all too common. How much water should we try & consume per day?

CH: Our fluid intake needs to increase when we are pregnant as our blood volume increases. We also need more fluid to create enough amniotic fluid, which is what our bub swims in. Drinking enough water can help with circulation and aid the nutrients we get from our diet to transfer to bub and remove toxins.

Staying adequately hydrated will help with many pregnancy symptoms such as cramps, constipation and headaches. The best way to make sure we are drinking enough water is to monitor the colour of our wee. A pale yellow is what we're aiming for.

As a general guide, 3L of water per day is a healthy amount – remembering that your cup of tea, soup, the water in your smoothie etc. can count towards your total intake. Get a good-looking water bottle with a straw! This will encourage you to drink throughout the day & it'll come in handy for labour and the breastfeeding thirst too!

Q. Foods to eat when suffering from constipation?

CH: Constipation is a very common pregnancy symptom so don't feel alone if you're struggling with this.

To avoid or help treat constipation and to reduce the likelihood of developing haemorrhoids we need to ensure we are consuming enough fluids and fibre. If we only increase the amount of fibre and not our fluid consumption as well, this can exacerbate constipation. So do your best to drink at least 3L of water per day.

High fibre foods include – chia seeds, whole fruits and vegetables, legumes, coconut, dates, prunes, nuts, wholegrains such as oats, quinoa, brown rice & rye bread.

Other things that can help with constipation include moving more, sitting correctly on the toilet (mimic a squat by using a step to have your knees above hips), eating more fat (fat lubricates the intestines and stimulates the release of bile which then stimulates contractions of the colon), eating fermented foods and/or considering a pregnancy safe probiotic supplement.

Q. Caro, are there particular foods that may induce labour? Is talk of eating dates true?

CH: There is some (weak) evidence to suggest that consumption of dates could induce natural labour, increase the rate of cervical dilation and may shorten labour. However dates also contain very high amounts of sugar and overconsumption may increase blood sugar levels for both mum and bub. This isn't a great thing. If you do want to eat more dates in the lead up to birth, I would encourage people to do so after eating protein to relieve the blood sugar spike.

Again there is some (very weak) evidence that drinking raspberry leaf tea can help to strengthen and tone the uterus for labour, decrease labour time and reduce the need for birthing interventions. Raspberry leaf tea is also a safe tea to drink during pregnancy and it's a good source of vitamin C, minerals & antioxidants. Be warned, it's an acquired taste.

Some women will find the ceremonial aspect of eating things like dates & consuming raspberry tea before birth helps to calm them and give them a sense of control over what is to come. I think it's really comforting especially if you have gone over your due date & you're anxious for baby to come. Just keep in mind that there is not enough evidence to draw any firm conclusions.

Q. Jumping forward to postpartum for a moment, what would you suggest women build into their diet after the birth?

CH: After birth is a very important time to focus on restoring your nutrient stores for the benefit of both your own health & the babies ... or if you want breastfeeding success. Nutrient needs are actually higher in breastfeeding mothers than what they were whilst pregnant!

It's helpful to think of it as if we're still growing the baby after the birth as we are their main source of food and therefore nutrients. As well as filling bubs tummy, it's important that we consume enough nutrient rich calories to help our bodies heal from pregnancy and birth.

If you continue eating the way you were during pregnancy (rich in vitamins, minerals, proteins, calcium, wholegrains, fibre etc), that's a good way to go about it. You could even expand the variety of foods you consume as food aversions and pregnancy nausea should have disappeared by now!

If you choose to breastfeed, you will need to consume more calories (approx. 500 more calories per day) for both milk supply & recovery, so make sure you listen to your body when it tells you it's hungry. Restricting your diet by consuming less food can result in breastmilk supply issues.

When the baby arrives, it can be hard to find the time to prepare good quality meals, I'd suggest preplanning prior to your due date (think – lots of freezer meals), and if someone offers to cook & deliver you a meal, say yes! Finally, make sure you have easy 'grab and go' snacks ready for when the hunger suddenly hits. Breastfeeding is likely to give your appetite a huge spike!

Q. What kinds of food should we look too in terms of postpartum recovery?

* Foods high in iron – such as meals with slow cooked meats. They're delicious and easy to digest.
* Foods high in omega 3s – fatty fish, eggs, poultry, beef.
* Warming & nutrient packed foods – think soups, slow cooked stews, Dahl, curries with lots of spices.
* Cooked vegetables – cooked veggies are much easier to digest compared to raw. Add lots of extra veggies to as many meals as possible i.e. stews, Dahl, curries, & soups.
* Cooked grains such as oats & rice.
* Bone broth – if you don't make your own there are lots of good quality bone broth products available to purchase.
* Lots of warming drinks and herbal teas – lactation teas, hot cacao and turmeric lattes are great!

There is a big emphasis on food that is 'warming' and food that is 'well-cooked' above. This is because your body will find it much easier to absorb the calories & the nutrients when food is prepared in this way, making it hugely beneficial for postpartum recovery.

Q. Important tips if you are a Vegan or Vegetarian?

CH: If you are vegan or vegetarian it can be more challenging to meet your nutritional needs during pregnancy. For this reason, I would **highly** encourage all vegan & vegetarians to work with a nutritionist or a dietician to ensure you are comfortably meeting your macro-nutrient needs (i.e. carbohydrates, protein, and fats) and your micro-nutrient needs (i.e. vitamins and minerals).

I'd imagine that in most cases both supplements & a consolidated meal plan would be required to keep you & the baby thriving. For vegans in particular, I'd encourage an open mind in terms of potentially expanding your dietary preferences over the 9 months to include some animal products. Of course this is my opinion only.

I've included some general considerations below but like anything else, before working anything into your diet or making any changes to your existing diet (especially if it's been planned by a dietician or nutritionist), always consult your health practitioner first or someone who knows your body & your pregnancy very well.

* Look into an algae based DHA supplement
* If you're vegetarian – eat full-fat dairy products such as yoghurt, cheese & kefir. Increase your intake of eggs (aim for 2 per day). Eggs are a nutrient powerhouse and will help you get closer to meeting your nutrient needs in terms of DHA, B12, vitamin A, choline etc.
* It's very important to look into a high quality prenatal vitamin that includes B12, iron and zinc. These are examples of the nutrients that are near impossible to get adequate amounts of when following a strict vegan diet.
* Consume lots of high quality wholegrains, legumes, nuts and seeds. It can be beneficial to consider soaking them before eating to maximise the nutrients absorbed. Grains, legumes, nuts and seeds contain phytic acid which inhibits mineral absorption in the body. Soaking them will lower the level of phytic acid, allowing greater absorption of minerals such as zinc, calcium, iron and magnesium.

Whole-wheat sourdough bread is the best bread choice in terms of maximising mineral absorption due to the bread's fermentation process.

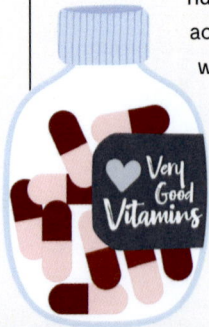

❤ Very Good Vitamins

PLEASE NOTE: Why have we not included a subsection to cover the Pescatarian diet? People who choose to follow a Pescatarian diet 'should' be able to derive sufficient nutrient levels during their pregnancy, if they include foods such as dairy and eggs in their diet.

I've read and re-read this chapter so many times as Caro's input changes the way you perceive a meal during pregnancy Food is fuel! It's not only filling and comforting – it's health inducing & energising and it grows the baby!

Some other noteworthy resources that cover health & nutrients during both pregnancy and postpartum (and the baby days!), are:

* *Village For A Mumma* by Leila Armour
* *The First 40 Days* by Heng Ou with Amely Greeven and Marisa Belger
* *Real Food in Gestational Diabetes* by Lily Nichols
* *Boob To Food* by Luka McCabe ... a goodie to buy as you prepare for baby. The book covers amazing content about the transition to solids! Note: Stock up on bibs & flannels.
* *Life After Birth* by Vaughne Geary and Jessica Prescott
* *How To Be Well* by Dr Karen Coates and Sharon Kolkka (not specific to pregnancy & postpartum but women's wellness in general)
* *The Postnatal Depletion Cure* by Dr Oscar Serrallach (best for postpartum)

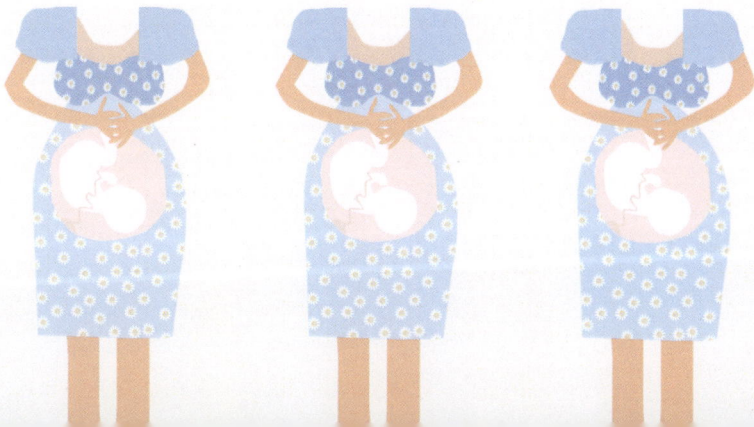

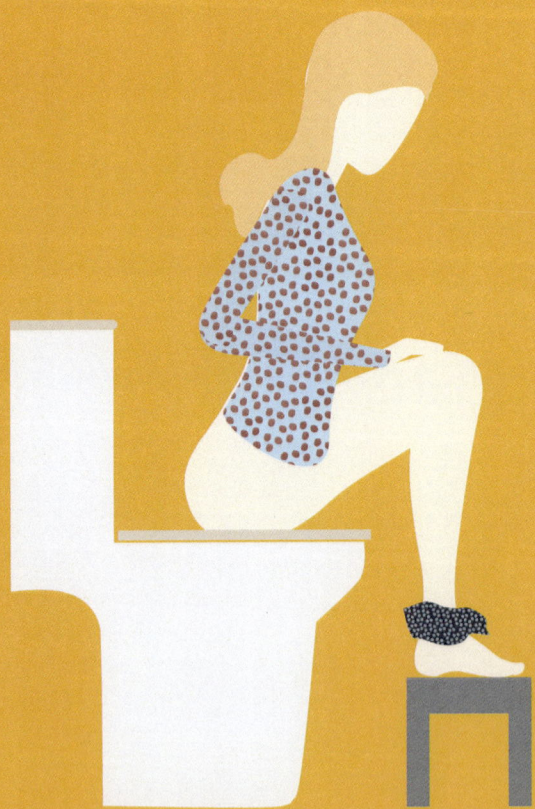

AVOIDING HAEMORRHOIDS • AVOIDING HAEMORRHOIDS

AVOIDING HAEMORRHOIDS • AVOIDING HAEMORRHOIDS

AVOIDING HAEMORRHOIDS

AVOIDING HAEMORRHOIDS • AVOIDING HAEMORRHOIDS

AVOIDING HAEMORRHOIDS • AVOIDING HAEMORRHOIDS

Maintaining healthy iron levels during pregnancy & in the lead up to birth is very important. For those with low iron levels, it's not uncommon if you're advised to take a daily iron supplement. I am one of those lucky folk. As this is a book you can't tell – but I use the term lucky with emphatic sarcasm. Why?

A common side of taking iron supplements is constipation (and black stools … how lovely!) … and what can follow persistent constipation is the arrival of Haemorrhoids. Not always, but sometimes. For anyone unsure about what a Haemorrhoid is, it's a swollen vessel around your rectum which can be either internal or external. They can be quite uncomfortable when you walk, sit or squat & they can bleed when you go to the loo. Again, how lovely!

Below are some tips to help with constipation & therefore prevent Haemorrhoids:

1. Drink plenty of water. Lots & lots of water especially if you're breastfeeding. A good idea is to get organised and buy yourself a big water bottle (1-2litres), before delivering. As you are so often sitting down with a baby glued to you in the early days, having a good water supply within arms reach is helpful.

2. Eat fresh! Eat lots of nutrient rich foods, full of fibre goodness. Fruit, veggies, nuts & seeds, dried fruit, wholegrain bread … the lot!

3. When you feel the need to go, GO! Don't ignore the urge as it'll only exacerbate the issue.

4. Stool softeners can be very helpful, especially if you're battling a Haemorrhoid. Much like their name, they'll soften the poop making it easier & perhaps faster to pass. *Easier & faster* are two words we like after labour.

5. Look into probiotics. Some of the delicious yogurts on the market can do wonders in terms of creating movement. Yogurts with probiotic strains can very positively support the digestive system by maintaining a balanced gut microbiota. In a nutshell, they can help to improve regularity.

You could also look into a probiotic supplement however it's highly recommended to check anything with your GP, midwife or maternal health nurse prior. A word of warning, it's best to stay clear of laxatives from the pharmacy or supermarket. If you're tempted for quick relief, I urge you to seek medical advice from your local health practitioner being buying or taking anything. Baby's health before a poop. Fair?

The above list is actually an extract from *AFTERWARDS*, my first book covering the topics of postpartum. So what about dealing with constipation and Haemorrhoids while you're pregnant? Firstly, I assume there are women reading who might fear pushing "too hard", in case they accidentally push their baby right? OR go into early labour?

If this sounds familiar, don't fret. You're not the only one thinking it. To ease your fear however & to bring about an easier poop, by all means peruse through the tips on the next page.

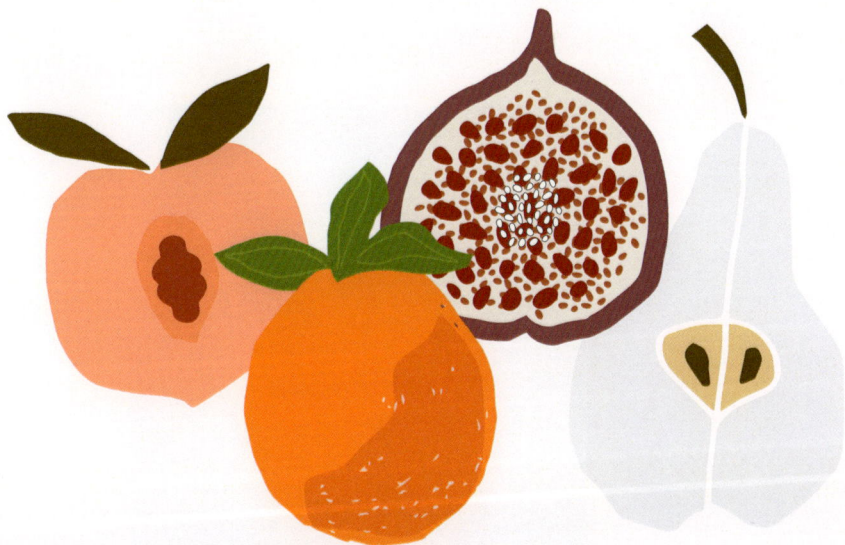

HELP EASE THE POOP

✳ **Posture:** Using a footstool, keep your knees higher than your hips & lean forwards as you make the "mooooo" sound. You'll feel your abdomen expand and some added pressure downwards in the rectum & anus which will assist with your bowel movement.

✳ **Eat Strategically:** Help your digestion system by making some easy-to-digest foods such as nutrient rich smoothies & soups. Sprinkling some additional fibre such as LSA or psyllium husk might be a nice idea.

✳ **Don't Over Do It:** If you're pushing with no relief, it's probably best to stop trying. You need to think about your pelvic floor here & you'll want to avoid causing a Haemorrhoid. Up the fluids, try & go for a slow walk and load up on fibre rich food. Think prunes, fresh Medjool dates, fruit toast, chia pods, fresh salads and leafy greens. Maybe even throw in a few glasses of Metamucil during the day.

✳ **If You Can, Get Moving:** Exercise (slow walks, swimming, some gentle squats, yoga), can help to create movement in the bowel and/or relieve constipation by lessening the time it takes food to move through your large intestine. This can reduce the amount of water your body absorbs from the stool i.e. softening your poops (charming right?!). Hard poops that are also dry will be much harder and more uncomfortable to pass. If you're open to it (and physically able), practicing gentle yoga is another way to encourage your bowels to get movin'. Particular yoga poses can massage the digestive tract and help to move stool through your intestines. Yoga usually includes lots of twists however, so make sure to check everything with a professional first as you want to protect your abdomen & of course, your baby!

May your tooshies remain peachy!

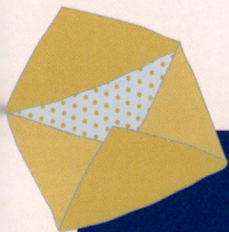

A Letter to Her Pregnant Self

FROM JESSIE

This mother, Jess, has experienced the heartache of miscarriage. She has so fearlessly healed & since birthed two dazzling little boys. Writing to her pregnant self after enduring such heavy loss, Jess delivers an artwork of words that mirror the warmth of a soul mate. For all other women who worry their pregnancy will be haunted by the bruise left from past loss. Here, Jess gently offers her understanding and support. You'll never be alone.

Dear me,

Congratulations! You are pregnant!

I know this moment feels bittersweet. You are staring at the test with tears streaming down your face. You are not sure if they are happy or sad.

You are still reeling from the loss of your last baby, still dealing with the trauma that came with it. You are allowed to grieve the child you felt you were promised.

That positive line feels like dejavu. You've learnt the hard way that life can be cruel.

Last time you had already told your partner the news that'd change your lives together, forever. You'd surprised your family, you had posted the social media announcement, you had held the ultrasound pictures. You bought an extra Christmas stocking. You've done it all before and ... and last time you felt like you let everyone down.

This moment, the one you've waited so desperately for, now feels tainted with that memory. The memory of what you have lost before.

I'm here to tell you that everything you are feeling is OK. Learning to once again trust the body, the body that has let you down will be hard. All pregnancies are different. This time around you will experience new symptoms, ones that you never expected.

You see, with every subsequent pregnancy your hormones build and things intensify. Your body is doing an amazing job as it relearns how to 'get back on the horse'. You are too. You and your body are one don't forget ... even though it might not seem like it right now.

I know that a part of you has had to disassociate your mind and body in order to get through child loss ... and to survive. You may not want to forgive it so soon. After all, who else can you blame for that dreadful loss?

This time, it'll be hard, I won't lie to you. You might be scared at each ultrasound as you wait with baited breath for the technician to tell you there's no heartbeat. You'll expect the worse and that is ok.

There will forever be a feeling at the pit of your stomach, the same place where your beautiful baby now grows. The feeling is a sort of dread that may not subside until the 20 week mark, or maybe even until your baby is in your arms. You'll lay awake at 4am playing out awful scenarios over & over in your head. You'll keep referring to post-birth life with the caveat 'if we are lucky enough to keep this one,' as if that if you say anything else you might jinx or curse yourself.

You might be envious of other pregnant women going through this for the first time. You'll watch them in waiting rooms in a blissful haze, drinking that awful glucose drink and placating you with questions you don't want to answer. These women have the oh so sweet gift of naivety. You, on the hand, know the dangers that lurk at every stage of a pregnancy.

You are forever changed.

Hindsight is a wonderful thing and here's why. I want to tell you why losing your last baby was beautiful ... bear with me.

People always talk about the 'miracle of life'. This holds a new meaning for you now.

With the swift and searing blows of grief, you'll be gifted a new lens for the world you live in.

You won't take this blessing for granted. Your capacity for empathy will grow tenfold. You will never ask another woman if she wants kids or if she wants another baby. You have a new found sensitivity to these things. It will be noticed and appreciated.

Grief will outshine joy for a little while. Death feels too near, an omnipresent threat. Motherhood is a shedding of skin and a growing of anew, just like a snake. One day, your new baby will be in your arms and that skin will still be visible, still nearby ... but it will be separate from you. It will no longer cover you in fear or constrict you with its stronghold on all the happiness you should be feeling.

The baby you now grow. When he arrives he will scream at the top of his lungs and it will be the greatest noise you've ever heard. He will cry as he leaves your body because that is where has been safe all this time. You can be sure of that now. He is here for real. Now you can believe it. That baby will look for your breast and into your eyes. He will meet the people you love. He will be held, rocked, carried, fed. Soon he will start walking. And talking. You will revel in his magic.

And one day in a moment you least expect, when he's running along the beach collecting rocks you'll be reminded of what you went through.

And instead of crying, you will smile.

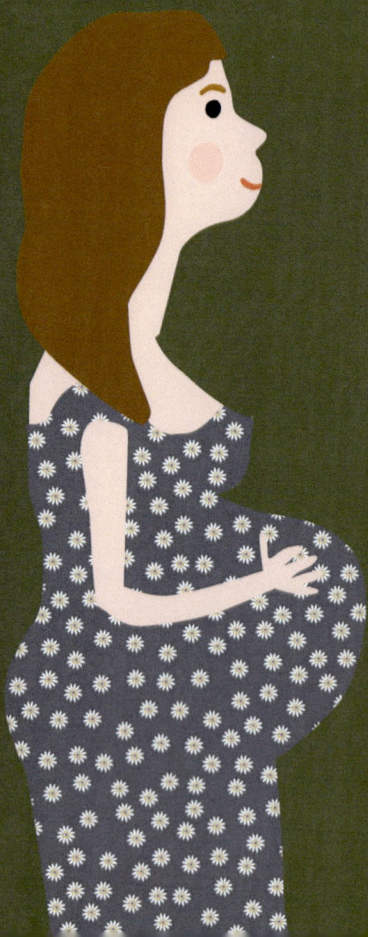

GESTATIONAL DIABETES

Let's start this chapter by talking about:

THE GLUCOSE TEST

What a bag of dicks this test is.

First of all, fasting for a whole day is horrendous when you're expecting. Depriving an irritable & nauseated pregnant lass of food is like depriving a marathon runner of water after their race. It's cruel.

We. Need. Snacks. People.

Three blood tests in three hours, on an empty belly is one thing. Having to drink 300mls of what can only be described as Elmo's morning syrup (i.e. thick, lukewarm glucose liquid), is another. The glucose liquid has to be consumed in the space of 5 minutes. Ughhh. While this may sound *easy-ish*, it ain't. Every sip gets thicker. And sweeter. And more aggressive. As your belly swells with the relentless onslaught of sugar, the waves of sea sickness roll in. *Ooft*. Tis a challenge to say the least.

Women have always complained about this test (which seems a little crazy considering they have the big show ahead, i.e. *birth*), but it is for good reason. The Glucose Test really does make you want to crawl under the couch and hide. I was SO nervous about it during my first pregnancy, I boycotted the test all together. Word of advice ladies, DO NOT FOLLOW SUIT! I am a good example of what NOT to do.

Gestational Diabetes (GD) is not a joke! And worryingly, it doesn't present any warning symptoms, which means the only way to pick it up, is to undergo this test. If you do contract GD and it's left untreated, it can lead to serious health implications for both you and your baby. So mothers-to-be, roll up your sleeves & bottoms up! It's go time.

Shall we learn more about Gestational Diabetes? I think so.

To preface, if you'd prefer a longer and more detailed insight into GD, I can highly recommend a podcast episode by one of my favourite mum duo's, Beyond The Bump, entitled *'Can Anyone Get Gestational Diabetes with Dr Timmy'*. It's a great listen that covers all aspects of GD and a huge list of FAQ's by mums alike. For here and now however, let's cover the basics.

TO NOTE: The below information is sourced from resources such as Diabetes Australia. Remember readers, I am not medically trained nor am I here to provide medical advice or make specific claims. I am simply here to make sure you understand the risks of GD and to make sure you don't chicken out of the test, like I did.

TO NOTE (AGAIN): I did do the test for my second pregnancy. High Five.

GD is a form of diabetes that occurs during pregnancy only, hence the use of the term 'gestational'. Post birth & in *most* cases, GD will dissipate – however there is a percentage of women who will go onto have high blood glucose levels after baby is born. These women should seek further medical advice for monitoring. Your GP is the first port of call when in doubt.

The Glucose Test is required around week 24. Hopefully by this stage your nausea and morning sickness will be well and truly done. If not, make sure you ask to have the test first thing in the morning. If you can get it over & done with asap in the morning, you can then load up on a comforting breaky around mid morning & save your belly from enduring another minute of illness.

As mentioned, the test includes 3 consecutive blood tests with an hour or so in between each. Given you're unable to eat for a quite sometime beforehand, many women vomit after drinking the syrup ... so best to take a spare top just in case.

How does the test work? It examines how your body digests glucose.

IS GESTATIONAL DIABETES COMMON?

It is common enough to be considered *likely*.

It may be best to answer this question by saying that under the diabetes umbrella, GD is the fastest growing category. In numbers, thousands of pregnant woman are diagnosed with GD, so please get yourself tested. The test may not be an enjoyable experience but as GD doesn't present symptoms, it can go unnoticed & undiagnosed. This then introduces risks for both mum & baby.

WHAT CAUSES GESTATIONAL DIABETES?

During pregnancy, a woman's placenta produces hormones that are required to feed & nurture the bub. As well as these hormones helping with bub's physical development, in the later stages of pregnancy the hormones (such as estrogen, cortisol & human placental lactogen) can start to block or resist a woman's insulin. This is not ideal as the need for insulin during pregnancy can be 2 to 3 times higher than usual.

Quick Interruption: *What is insulin? (And this is not a silly question by-the-by... I had no idea either before becoming pregnant!)*

Firstly, Insulin is a hormone. It's created by the body's pancreas, which is the gland that sits behind your stomach, in your upper abdomen. In simple terms your pancreas helps the digestion system by creating enzymes & hormones (one of which is, of course, insulin). The enzymes break down starches, sugars & fats (aka the rapid influx of the 1st Trimesters hot pastry & sweet sugar binges), and at all times the Insulin regulates the amount of glucose (which is a type of sugar) in your bloodstream.

If the level of sugar in your bloodstream is too high, you may experience hyperglycaemia. If too low, you may experience hypoglycaemia. Both of which are not ideal and should be very carefully monitored (whether pregnant or not).

When you eat, your body metabolises the consumed carbohydrates (i.e. food) and breaks it down into sugar molecules, including glucose. When this happens, your body's blood glucose level will rise, which then signals your pancreas to release Insulin. Insulin then helps the body store these sugars for later when your body needs energy. Storage takes place in your muscles and/or your liver. Got all that?! How incredible is the human body!

If your body does not release Insulin & you suffer from Insulin resistance, your blood sugar levels can surpass a healthy level and lead to negative health implications. In the case of a pregnant women, these implications can affect both mother & child.

According to *Pregnancy, Birth & Baby* online in 2022, 1 in 8 pregnant women will be diagnosed with (GD), between 24 and 28 weeks.

WHY DO PREGNANT WOMEN GET GESTATIONAL DIABETES?

Generally speaking, when you're pregnant your blood sugar levels are likely to be higher than when you're not pregnant. Your body should be able to create and deliver Insulin sufficiently, however, during pregnancy the chances of it failing to do so are much higher. If failure occurs, this can lead to GD.

There is an old myth that only overweight people inherit diabetes. Why? Obesity (or when your BMI is above 30) can cause increased levels of fatty acids and inflammation in the body, which lends itself to Insulin resistance. While pregnant women are certainly not obese, they are carrying additional weight which can affect their blood sugar levels.

To reduce your chances of GD, maintaining a clean & balanced diet is essential, as is exercise. Eating a balance of protein, multigrains and fruit & veg every day is a great start. Load up on healthy fats such as omega 3's, eggs, nuts, avocado and pasteurised diary*, and limit your intake of processed food.

Pasteurised Dairy refers to cheese & milk products that have undergone a process where they are heated to a particular temperature to kill any harmful bacteria or organisms including E.coli, Salmonella, Listeria. *Unpasteurised Dairy* refers to foods like cheese & milk that have not undergone this heating process. Examples of Unpasteurised Dairy includes milk straight from a cow and a variety of popular soft cheeses … brie, camembert, gorgonzola and other blue vein cheeses.

We digress. Back to the subject of GD!

Roughly 10-20% of women diagnosed with GD will require Insulin injections until the birth. These same women will also need to maintain a stricter diet & do whatever is possible to incorporate movement into their day, even if it's a daily waddle to the shops.

The good news? *Most* of the time GD should pass when the baby is born and as your body returns to its pre-baby functions. To be sure, you should get a test at your 6 week check up to ensure you're back in the safe zone.

CAN YOU PREVENT GESTATIONAL DIABETES?

Some cases of GD are genetic. If it is genetic in your case, it's unlikely you will be able to bypass the diagnosis. With this in mind, continue doing whatever you can to prioritise a healthy diet & exercise regime. The multifaceted benefits of good health are always worth prioritising.

Where possible, take the stairs instead of the lift or walk to the cafe or grocery store instead of driving. Try to curb the naughty cravings with solid tactics. It's all about *the play*. And the play is? To Play Defence mumma.

Instead of purchasing a two litre bucket of ice cream & going rogue with your spoon after dinner, why not purchase a box of individual frozen yogurts? Instead of guzzling a can of Sprite or Coke, find a pregnancy safe collagen, probiotic or vitamin supplement to pimp your soda water. When you want … sorry, when you *need*… to eat a block of chocolate, smear some Nutella onto grainy toast. There are always ways!

GD can not only affect the pregnant woman but it can also affect the darling unborn child. Without inciting unnecessary fear or panic here, it is important to point out that if GD is left undiagnosed or untreated, it can lead to premature birth, birthing a larger baby (meaning there is a higher risk of intervention such as the need for a Caesarean delivery), miscarriage or stillbirth.

Get the test. Do the work. And keep GD at bay. Make sure to talk openly to your GP and ask as many questions as you have. The more you know, the better.

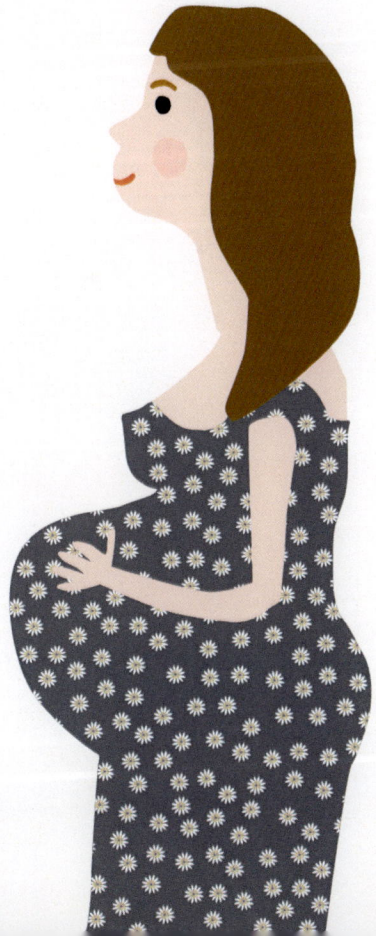

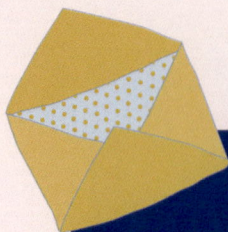

A Letter to Readers

FROM GEORGIE

Like most pregnant women I was booking into scans and appointments as my OB instructed. She said this next one was going to be a 2 hour blood test so, '*make sure you book in first thing in the morning as you have to fast beforehand. And take a book or your laptop to keep you occupied because the test lasts 2 hours.*'

As she said … I did.

Blissfully naïve to what I was being tested for I walked in and was handed 'the sweet drink' … which is essentially pure glucose.

People had warned me that this 'sweet drink' was disgusting, to the point they got shivers just talking about it.

To the contrary I semi-enjoyed the drink. It tasted like thick-flat lemonade. Not overly enjoyably but not terrible. The 3 other pregnant women in the waiting room looked physically ill after drinking theirs. One of the women held a vomit bag and tried desperately not to spew. If she did, she would have to come another day and start it all over again – not ideal. I believe there are other ways to test for GD but this is the most common.

On my way home I called my friend who'd had gestational diabetes during pregnancy and I asked her, ' What's all the fuss about? It's not that bad …?' She said that's what she had also thought and… (perhaps it's an old wives tale), but as she semi-enjoyed the drink like I did… maybe it was likely I have GD as well?

Sure enough, the next day my OB called to say that I did have GD & she was sending me to a nutritionist and diabetes specialist.

I asked her … so what is GD?

My OB explained that the condition is diagnosed during pregnancy (hence 'gestational') and it affects how you use and break down sugar.

GD can causes high blood sugar and can affect your babies heath and generally produces 'bigger babies'. However, you can control GD predominantly by healthy eating and exercise and if deemed necessary ... by medication.

I was able to control mine by healthy eating and regular exercise (without medication) ... I did Pilates 2-3 times a week and would do a lap around the block after dinner (the last thing you feel like doing when pregnant). When you have GD you get a 'pricker' and strips to prick and test your blood sugar levels 4 times a day for the remainder of your pregnancy. I'm not going to lie .... your fingers get sore and sensitive and you soon find yourself searching for the 'least sore' fingertip to prick.

I found pricking my fingers quite confronting for the first few days but one week in and it was second nature and not a big deal!

There are all sorts of stats and medical advise you get bombarded with once you know you have GD but what I can say from my experience ... is that even though the ONE THING you look forward to the most when you are pregnant is eating whatever you like!!! ... and that becomes NOT the case for women with GD ... in hindsight I have to say that having gestational diabetes was an absolute **blessing** in disguise.

I was forced to eat really well and felt very strong and healthy throughout my pregnancy. I believe my energy levels were far better to what they would have been had I continued to eat copious Tim Tams and croissants. And the **best BEST** part was my recovery post birth. It was a very fast recovery and my body 'bounced back' within weeks. My other friends who have have had GD during their pregnancy have all said the same thing.

The strangest thing about GD is that you may have it in one pregnancy but not the next.. For those reading, if like me you have GD... fear not... because the second you have that beautiful baby.... you can go back to eating whatever you want!!!

Cue the ice cream!

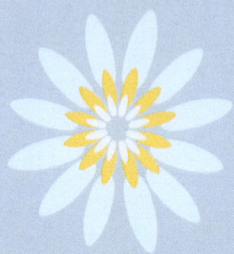

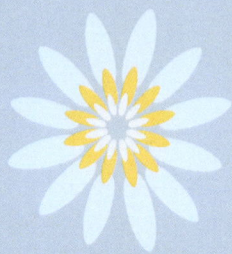

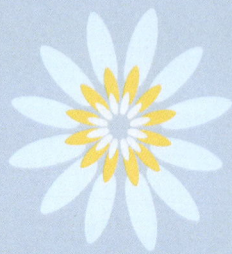

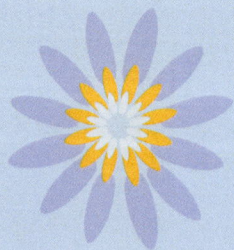

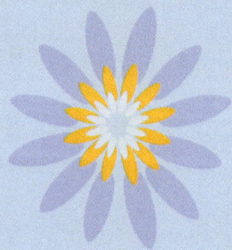

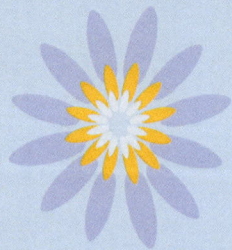

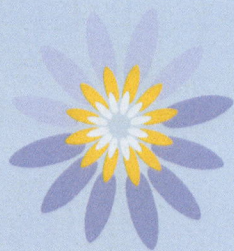

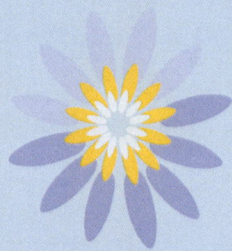

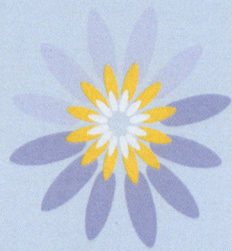

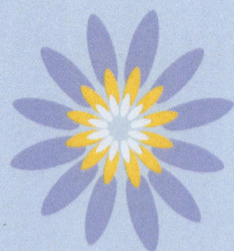

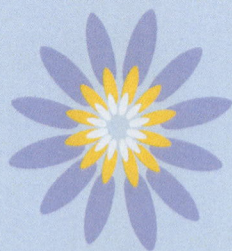

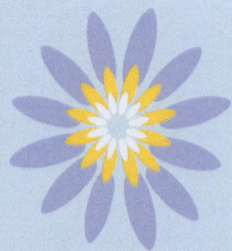

THE DARLING DOULA

OH DARLING DOULA. WHAT ARE YOU? WHO ARE YOU? WHERE ARE YOU?! All good questions if you ask me! Personally I didn't have a Doula for either baby however if I had a third bub, I would invest in a Doula for sure! Why? Growing a baby, birthing a baby, raising a baby while trying to adjust, heal, survive – is tiring. In many, many different ways.

While I had an incredible support system and a wonderful partner (my husband & the father of my boys), having a Doula would be similar to having a 'spiritual friend' holding your hand from go-to-woe. A third party who exists to bring you comfort, empathy & warmth. Sound nice? I think so.

Postpartum doula Tiffany Smith-Shiels aka The Ritual Doula (@tiff_theritualdoula) has graciously leant her time & light to answer the many wonders you may have.

Q. **What is a Doula & where did the concept originate from?**

TS: The word "doula" comes from ancient Greek, meaning **"a woman who serves"** or "woman servant". In regards to a postpartum doula I like to refer to it as mothering the mother.

Today, "doula" refers to a person trained to provide emotional, physical and informational support to women throughout their pregnancy, birth and the early postpartum period.

A postpartum doula is employed to provide guidance and support to the mother of a newborn baby.

Q. **What is a complete myth about Doulas – is far from true?**

TS: That we are somewhat medically trained, which we are not.
That we are here to be the role of the partner ... we are not – we are EXTRA support for the birthing person.

Q. **Why would one opt for a Doula?**

TS: Because the fourth trimester is totally underrated about how much support is needed and if you are aware of this then investing in postpartum care would be an absolute priority. I'm sure that no mother has ever said they had too much postpartum support! Hehe

Q. When does the Doula '"enter & exit" in terms of the pregnancy, birth & postpartum timeline?

TS: For postpartum, the window can be from day one post birth to 2 months on average BUT postpartum is forever. So really for as long as any mother needs support.

Q. Is a Doula a qualified medical professional?

TS: No we are not.

Q. What training does a Doula typically have?

TS: Depending on level/type of doula it can range from a 3 month online course to years of training.

Q. How much does a Doula usually cost?

TS: Again, depending on offerings and packages. It can range from on average one visit on online consultation of $200 to $5,000 packages.

Q. *"I would love a Doula however my partner thinks it would be invasive during such an intimate family time."* What would you say to this?

TS: Totally understandable. Coming into a home at SUCH a raw, intimate and vulnerable time I can see why a partner could say this. I feel such honour to be entering your home in this time, its' not something I take lightly. However I feel I navigate my visits to be as invisible as possible. Also I'm not a guest. I am a supportive staff member in the postpartum window. I'd repeat 'when has a birthing person ever said that they received too much support?'. If mum feels that a PP doula is going to nourish, hold and support her then partner hopefully hears and lets us in!

Q. What are some things no one knows about Doula's?

TS: That doulas have been around since the beginning of time. Despite this I'm constantly explaining what I do as a vocation – as people seem to think it's a new role. Not that I mind. The more people know the better!

Q. Why have you chosen to become a Doula?

TS: A number of reasons. I was held and supported wonderfully when I experienced pregnancy loss. I'll never forget it. So I wanted to offer this service to all spectrums of postpartum. I love all things about women centred care.. and I feel that in the modern world we have lost the village. I hope my visits I bring a one woman village feel .

Q. Your advice to all expecting Mummas?

TS: Organise or get friend/relative/postpartum doula to organise you a meal train!

I have so much respect for the role of a Doula. Everything that comes with growing & birthing a baby, plus nurturing that baby & your body is a lot to take on. The days can feel heavy as the magnitude of needs tugs on your arms, your boobs, your tired eyes, your hands & your heart. A Doula offers empathetic support. A Doula can feed you, tend to your aching body & hold your darling child as you take the time to rest, recover or simply make some Vegemite toast before diving into the next series of a trashy soap.

Even if you don't think you're a "Doula" person ..... do some reading first. They don't replace the medical support team needed for your pregnancy, they simply offer a new layer to life. And my word, that layer is comforting and delicious!

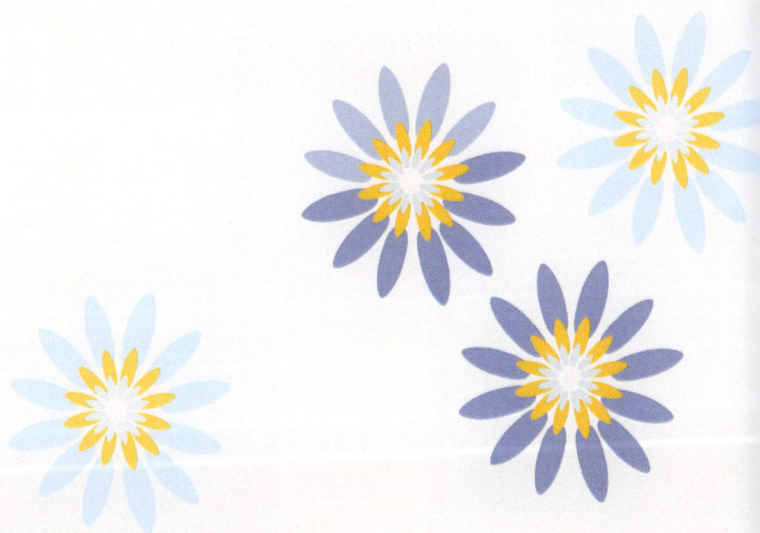

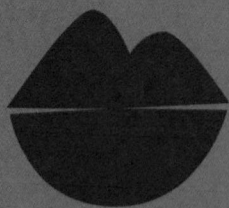

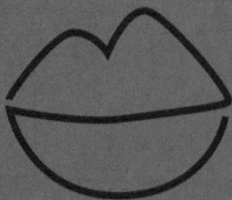

SEX ● SEX ● SEX ● SEX ● SEX ● SEX

SEX ● SEX ● SEX ● SEX ● SEX ● SEX

SEX ● SEX ● SEX ● SEX ● SEX ● SEX

SEX

SEX ● SEX ● SEX ● SEX ● SEX ● SEX

When you're carrying some extra kilograms, feeling a little bloated or you are hugely nauseated. When your sciatic nerve is keeping you up all night or you're a tad gassy or backed up ... you know what I think sounds bloody fantastic? Sex.

HA. HA.

But in all seriousness – a lot of women will crave sex more than usual during their pregnancy, despite the onslaught of fatigue & aches. Not all women, but it's definitely not uncommon to experience surges in your sex drive while carrying a baby, so if that includes you, don't fight it! Lean into ladies. Enjoy it!

Sex during pregnancy, well what a ride this will be. As mentioned, you'll either crave it and experience randier moods than usual – due to the hormonal shifts in your body – or, on the flip side you may feel as though you'd rather your partner pack up and head off camping for 9 months as you find yourself experiencing a complete disinterest in any form of intimacy. Partners, don't take this personally. Instead, please come home with treats and then allow a radius of at least 1m from your pregnant partner at all times unless instructed otherwise.

Even if you are not quite 'craving' sex or 'dreading' sex, there is a wide spectrum of feelings in between ... and it could change by the week, by the day, by the hour. Just like newborns, pregnancy doesn't offer much predictability. After two pregnancies, I can safely say that the feelings around sex can be vastly different for each pregnancy. Don't categorise yourself too soon. Go with the flow.

The most important take-home before we take a deep dive into the subject of sex during pregnancy, with our brilliant resident sexologist – while you are pregnant (and to be honest, ALWAYS in general), **you** are in control of **your** bedroom, **your** body, **your** needs & wants. Never let anyone or any emotion (such as guilt), persuade you to launch into a midweek romp if it's not what you feel like. Your body, mind & mood is preoccupied with something so much bigger than sex. Satisfying the needs of your partner is not your priority, ok mummas? After all, there are other ways they can relieve themselves should they find themselves wading in desperate waters. Right? Right!

If however, your sex drive has remained unchanged or if you notice it has increased & you're keen to kickstart some action between the sheets... let's talk!!!!

Let us peel back the layers to unveil Sex During Pregnancy.

So enough from me for now! Let's chat to the wonderful Aleeya Hachem, who is our experienced & wildly informative Sexologist and Fertility Counsellor. After reading this chapter, please do yourselves a favour & make sure to follow her at @great. sexpectations to continue learning. This magic individual is someone to keep close on your radar! Over to Aleeya!

AN INTRODUCTION FROM ALEEYA ...

'The idea of sex and pregnancy is often considered taboo, with society preferring to view these as separate mentalities. However, we are beginning to move away from this idea, with individuals and couples focusing on pleasure and a fulfilling sex life during the 9-10 months of pregnancy. It is important to note that the term sex isn't exclusive to sexual penetration alone (between heterosexual couples.) Rather, sex encompasses outercourse (external stimulation,) masturbation and more broadly – intimacy.

If you and/or your partner have any questions or concerns about your libido or sex in general during pregnancy you can always have a chat to your doctor, or more specifically a sexologist. No question is a dumb question, we are here to help you navigate this season of your life.'

Now! Shall we explore the many questions us gals are all wondering about? Yes we shall!

Q. Managing Our Libido During Pregnancy. Aleeya, talk to us about this concept!

AH: Navigating the ever-changing shifts in libido during pregnancy can be challenging, as each trimester is so unique in the way it affects our bodies.

The first trimester is often associated with bouts of nausea and extreme fatigue, so it's not surprising that the last thing on your mind is having sex. As the pregnancy progresses through to the second trimester, you may start to feel more like yourself again, which can cause a surge in libido for some. Additionally, the increased blood flow to pelvic region can increase sensation and pleasure. Throughout the third trimester, libido can fluctuate based on how you are feeling on any given day; some days you may be exhausted and others you may be ready to go.

Managing libido, whether it be high or low, requires constant communication with your partner. Your partner is not a mind reader, and they are not the one growing a human, so help them understand how you are feeling. As pregnancy continuously changes how you look and feel about your body, you and your partner will need to define what your new sexual boundaries are, particularly around safe sex practices in pregnancy.

If you don't feel up to penetrative sex, remove the pressure entirely and focus on intimacy in general with your partner. This can look different for every couple: a make out session, a foot rub on the couch, a dinner date or even rubbing your belly with beautiful body oil. Focusing on the things that bring you close to your partner can help you both to feel connected if you notice your libido is low.

There is great variability regarding libido in pregnancy – know whatever you are feeling at this very moment is normal!

Q. Nurturing your relationship during pregnancy is important as it may waiver in many directions, some of which might be slightly downhill. There are hormones circulating in your body, you each have tremendous change in

sight – *which will knowingly catapult you both into unfamiliar territory* – and you're all of sudden becoming a newer version of yourselves, parents-to-be. Aleeya, can you enlighten us with ways to ready our relationships for both the pregnancy and those early newborn days?

Pregnancy is a turbulent time: body changes, hormonal shifts, numerous health appointments and preparing for the arrival of a bub Whilst planning for the postpartum period is necessary, try to stay present and enjoy this time with your partner. If this is your first baby, it's some of the final moments of partnership before you become a family of three, which changes the dynamic of the relationship significantly. Schedule quality time together and prioritise those conversations about how you will navigate your relationship through the postpartum period.

Some conversations that can be useful to have during pregnancy:

* 'How can we effectively navigate our routine with a serious lack of sleep?'
* 'How can we prioritise intimacy each day?'
* 'What does the division of tasks in our household look like, and is this sustainable through changing phases?'

Q. Back to sex! Let's talk to the subject of body confidence as pregnancy can unveil a whole new shape! Some women will love it (myself included because finally I'm awarded boobs & hips from the anatomy god!), and other women will find themselves hugely uncomfortable in their changing skin.

It is inevitable that your body will change during pregnancy – it's undergoing rapid change from a physical perspective to allow your beautiful baby to grow. We are so used to having control of our bodies and pregnancy requires you to let go and surrender to the process. If your body confidence is low in pregnancy, you are certainly not alone. Some days you may feel great about your body and others, not so much.

Some practical tips on dealing with low body confidence during pregnancy include:

* Focusing on all the amazing things that your body is doing right now can help to shift mindset from what your body looks like to how it is functioning to serve you and baby
* Investing in what makes you feel sexy– could this be beautiful lingerie? Clothes that fit your changing body and hug your new curves? A mani/pedi or a blow wave? These are acts of self-care so consider this your permission to prioritise them.
* Look at pictures of pregnant women (either with or without clothes) to normalise the changing changes.. Pregnant women are beautiful, and sometimes seeing these images helps to highlight that you are just as beautiful too.

Pregnancy is a season, and there may be a day where you miss that beautiful bump.

Q. Myth or Fact?! Some sexual positions can help to naturally induce labor ?

While certain sex positions do not bring on labor per se, sexual intercourse can get things moving. This is because certain proteins found in semen cause the cervix to soften and thin out, leading to the onset of contractions. That doesn't mean that sex during pregnancy is likely to cause pre-term labor by any means, but if you are 40 weeks and well over it your doctor may prescribe sex to speed things along.

Q. Let's back up a few steps. Sex toys are so widely and comfortably celebrated these days, thanks to confident & encouraging women like yourself. Are sex toys safe during pregnancy?

Sex toys are safe during pregnancy and can work to enhance sensation during solo and/or partnered sex. A few things to note:

* Make sure that toys are cleaned thoroughly with toy cleaner or warm soapy water to avoid infection.
* Avoid toys that can cause air blowing into the vagina.
* If using toys anally, make sure they are thoroughly cleaned before inserting into the vagina.

✳ Although you may find yourself more 'wet' during pregnancy, don't be afraid to add that extra lube to make things more comfortable for you.

Q. How about masturbation. Safe during pregnancy?

Absolutely! The benefits of masturbation are endless, such as increased mood, pain relief, better sleep and to help lower stress. Increased blood flow to the pelvis and hormonal changes may lead to more intense orgasms also which can make it even more fun.

Certain stimulation that you found pleasurable before pregnancy may change as you progress through each trimester. Masturbation is a great way to learn about how you like to receive pleasure, which enables us to effectively communicate this to our partner during partnered sex.

Q. Are there any risks to be aware of regarding having sex during pregnancy?

Thankfully, none unless specifically stated by your health practitioner.

There are some sexually transmitted infections (STI's) that can be dangerous for developing babies, such as chlamydia, gonorrhoea, and HIV. It is important to use barrier method of contraception (such as condoms) if you are not in a monogamous relationship. If you think you could be at risk of these infections, please talk to your practitioner about appropriate testing.

Q. Ok let's get juicy! What positions might be more favourable or comfortable during pregnancy for our mummas-to-be?

In the first trimester, any sex position that you feel comfortable with is the best position for you. From 28 weeks, it is best to avoid positions where you are lying on your back or there is pressure on the belly, as this can restrict blood flow to the baby and cause you to feel faint.

Some of the best sex positions for pregnancy include:

* **Cowgirl or pregnant person on top** – can control depth of penetration and clitoral stimulation.
* **Side lying or spooning** – very comfortable and keeps the weight off your belly.
* **Doggy style or from behind** – can be on all fours or standing up. Make sure you rest against something to avoid fatigue.
* **Missionary** – try positioning yourself onto the end of the bed with your partner standing or holding themselves up.

Q. **Pandering to very sore & tender boobs is a huge part of the 9 month pregnancy adventure. Any tips or tricks to avoid discomfort during sex?**

Ah the breast changes during pregnancy. Tenderness and an increase in size can be quite the adjustment alongside a growing belly. Not only may you feel discomfort but leaking can sometimes occur during sex when you feel aroused, or your breasts are stimulated. This is because oxytocin (the 'love' hormone) is also responsible for causing the let-down reflex.

While your partner may find your 'new' breasts exciting, it's important to communicate if you don't want this area touched. Outlining this as a sexual boundary before sex can help avoid ruining the mood in the moment. For example, you could say 'I would prefer it if you don't touch my boobs this time, but I would love it if you could grab my thighs instead.'

Choose certain sex positions (such as side-lying or missionary) to take the pressure off the breasts and wear a bra or lingerie to cover the area if you feel self-conscious. There are some fantastic maternity/nursing lingerie brands that look beautiful while ensuring the health of the breast tissue.

Q. **What should women know and/or do if they notice bleeding or spotting during or after sex?**

Some spotting or a small amount of bleeding after sex during pregnancy is normal, as the cells in the cervix change and become more sensitive. Although it can be quite scary, spotting should subside within 24 hrs and become lighter. Use a pad or a panty liner until the bleeding subsides, rather than inserting a tampon. If you notice a large amount of blood, or bleeding increases in the following 24 hours call your doctor for further investigation.

Q. **If a woman's partner has fears around 'hurting the baby' or if a male partner is nervous to have sex in case he 'nudges the baby!'... how can we manage this concern?**

This is a very normal and valid concern! There is a misconception, particularly among partners, that sex can hurt the baby which can lead to fear or avoidance of sex during pregnancy. The amniotic sac keeps your baby warm and protected, and the baby is nowhere near the vaginal canal or the cervix during sex. They are also completely oblivious to sex in the womb – the only thing that they will feel is the rhythmic rocking, which is likely to lull them to sleep!

Be patient and understanding of your partner as you unpack any fears associated with sex in pregnancy. Sometimes hearing information about sex in pregnancy from your health practitioner can make your partner feel more at ease and provide them with further reassurance.

It's easy & natural to feel timid when it comes to matters surrounding sex! Especially during pregnancy when you're noticing changes to your body, your libido, your energy. Aleeya is a fabulous expert (and mother herself!) and I strongly urge you all to follow her @great.sexpectations to explore your curiosities, find advice, seek comfort and/or to simply enjoy her highly informative, inclusive, relatable and palatable content. In summary, pregnant women can of course have sex, crave sex and ENJOY sex!! And remember, sex is on YOUR terms!

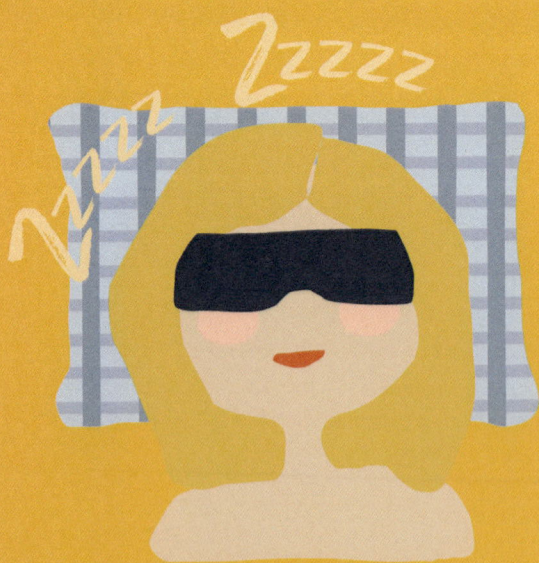

SLEEP

Sleep. What a scrumptious word sleep is. I can only imagine that every second person is giving you the following advice when they notice your pregnant belly, 'Sleep as MUCH as you can before the baby arrives! Because when they arrive ...' As irritating as the frequency of this advice becomes over time, there is truth to it. Personally, if I had my time again, I would have taken more time to be horizontal during my pregnancies...but we women are busy bees aren't we! So don't beat yourself up if you're not sleeping during the day. Enjoying some 'you time' can be just as sacred.

On the topic of sleep, it shouldn't be a shock to learn that clocking up consecutive hours of deep sleep is trickier when the baby comes along. Those little cuties just love to party in the wee hours! Prior to arriving at that point of life, perhaps some valuable information around how to prepare for the upcoming night feeds may help?

When I was pregnant for the first time, I always used to think, 'How the f**k does someone get up once or twice or three plus times EVERY night & still function the next day? HOW!'

Mirroring the awake hours of your nocturnal baby is quite a hideous task to be frank. Sure, your baby is sweet to cuddle in the early hours when they're warm & snug, but they are equally as cute between 9am and 5pm. Cuter in fact. The fact is that humans were not designed to be awake at 3am. We were designed to be under a warm blanket while dreaming & drooling on a pillow.

Mummas (and Daddas if you're reading!!), I am sorry to say, but it's just a matter of sucking it up & powering through. New babies must eat, so it's time to wake up & smell the sleep none of us are enjoying. On the bright side, as hard as it is to fathom, your body will adjust after a few weeks. I promise! Humans are exceptionally adaptable beings. And women in particular, we're superheroes.

So to help us prepare for what's coming & how to best cope/deal/survive ... we have the brilliant sleep consulting Francesca Kendall. Fran founded The Sleep Escape (@the.sleep.escape), which is a must read sleep guide for new babies. I've used it, loved it & swear by it! For the purpose of this book however, Fran has kindly turned her attention to the Mumma-bear-to-be. Below you'll find insights into many of the queries I imagine many of you will have (myself included!).

Q. **Fran welcome! To start off, are there ways women can prepare for their newborns feeding pattern before the birth?**

FK: It's good to be aware that an average baby (3.5kg and term) will feed every 3 hours overnight for the first few weeks. Some babies will stretch out their feeds more and others won't quite make 3 hours, but understanding that this is what your baby needs to meet their demand may help to ease a woman's fear around the frequency of the night feeds.

If you're bottle feeding expressed milk or formula, you will probably find the baby can do longer stretches as unlike breastfeeding, you will know & therefore have some control over how much they are getting at each feed.

Getting up 3 to 4 times overnight sounds terrible, however thankfully postpartum hormones help a lot! You'll be surprised how well you manage & adapt. Napping during the day is advised.

If you feel like the feeding has been established and you'd like your partner to help, my advice is to delegate them the late night feed (i.e. after 9pm) using a bottle. If you don't want to introduce a bottle however, ask your partner to bring bub to you for a feed & then they can take bub to burp and change so that your 'wake up' is as short as possible. You'll feel like a different person if you can get a good stretch of consecutive sleep during the first half of the night. On top of this, it's a nice way for your partner to bond with the baby.

Q. **For the feeds during the wee hours, where do you recommend women set up there feeding station? In bed? The nursery or living room?**

FK: This will differ as it'll depend on where you feel most comfortable feeding. Personally I preferred feeding in bed or in the nursery as everything I needed was close by i.e. the change table. Where you feed however, may also depend on your birth. If you're recovering from a cesarian, you may need to feed in bed.

A quick tip on feeding. Wherever I fed I'd always position a big bowl to collect the dirty equipment (bottles/pump parts etc). This made it really easy & efficient to transport it all into the kitchen for sterilising. A never ending job!

Q. Surrounding the feeding station, what helps to keep in reach?

FK: Designate a big bottle of water to your feeding station & ensure it stays there. Then grab another for when you are on the go. This way, you'll always be able to rehydrate mid-feed which is important. Allocating the job of keeping all bottles full is a good one for your partner to take care of. It's one less thing for you to think about!

For the night feel I recommend having a night-light close that you can use instead of turning on the main light or using your phone torch. The less bright you make it, the easier it'll be for you to fall back to sleep. The Sleep Escape's light & white noise machine is very handy as it can hang by the side of the bassinet making it easy to reach & find. You can buy these online.

Q. When feeding overnight, many mums tend to distract themselves with a phone, the TV or a Podcast. Is there a chance we'll overstimulate ourselves & find it harder to go back to sleep? OR do you think it's best for women to feed however keeps them sane?

FK: Scrolling on your phone is so natural these days. And it can feel like a necessary distraction to get through the night feeds. They can be long, particularly in the early days. My opinion is to do whatever gets you through this period. If you start to find it harder to fall back to sleep post feed, I'd definitely recommend putting your phone away or at the very least turning the brightness down to it's minimum.

Q. Regarding relationships, some partners opt to get up during the night with the mum to help. Is this support suggested? Or is it better to have at least one well rested parent?

FK: This is a personal preference. Personally, I didn't want my partner awake at the same time as bub as there wasn't much he could help me with. Having an unnecessarily tired partner the next day is not ideal, especially when they could be proactive & take care of the washing, cleaning and sterilising.

Having said this, of course there may be times when having your partner there as support is exceptionally helpful. If the baby isn't settling for example or if you're become tired or irritable, asking your partner to take over is a great solution. Babies will feed off your energy. If your partner is rested & calm, the bub may return to sleep sooner in their arms.

Q. If the partner feels guilty for NOT getting up during the night, how can they compensate?

FK: A good idea is to keep a To-Do list on the fridge listing everything that needs taking care of during the day. If your partner can get up & sort through the listed items throughout the day, your mental load will lighten and everyone will be happier. You'll find that not everything needs doing everyday however just knowing that someone else is keeping tabs on the many jobs around the house is very reassuring.

Q. Getting up in the dark & cold to find a crying or unsettled baby can feel quite depressing night after night. How do new mums protect their mental health?

FK: It's hard. Especially when you have just fallen into really deep sleep & wake to the cry of your baby night after night, week after week. Remembering that this period won't last forever is the key. It's an important phase of their growth, which is required so they can develop and thrive! As time goes on however, they will sleep, and so will you.

Q. We all hear about the 4 month sleep regression. For new mums, can you explain what this means and how they can best prepare?

FK: Yes! Newborns only have two stages of sleep; 'Stage 3' and 'Stage 4'. They spend 50% in each stage however around 3 or 4 months their sleep starts to re-organise itself. It's around now they begin to embrace the '4 Stage Method of Sleep' like adults.

The 'Stage 4' sleep i.e. REM sleep, becomes reduced to 25%, creating more room for Stages 1 and 2. This means the baby spends more time in a 'light sleep' phase, making them more susceptible to waking up. To manage the extent of how much this change affects them, implementing healthy sleep habits at this point can really help.

Healthy habits during the first 12 weeks can include:

* Creating a dark room for their day naps when you're at home (blackout blinds can help with this)
* Following their neurological awake windows. This will stop them going into the regression already overtired
* Giving them a bath before bed
* Introducing a book before bed, or a massage
* Following the same bed routine each night

Q. **We should be brutally realistic & acknowledge that some mothers will have babies who simply 'refuse' to sleep, or who suffer from colic or reflux issues. For mothers who worry they'll come across these issues, any advice?**

My advice would be to not worry about creating 'bad habits' until a rough patch has passed. If your baby needs to sleep on you for example i.e. in your arms or on your chest to receive restorative sleep, then do it! If they're suffering from colic or reflux, it's better to work with the babies preference to encourage sleep & prevent them becoming overtired.

If you find they sleep well in the pram or the carrier as opposed to the bassinet, I encourage it. Colic and reflux tends to subside around the 12 week mark, so after this you can start to help them learn to sleep independently. Just focus on getting through the tough period as best you can and worry about the rest later.

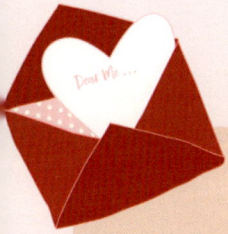

A Letter to Her Pregnant Self

FROM JESSICA

This mother defines resilience to the nth degree. Carrying her second daughter, she writes back in time to encourage feelings of hope, to offer reassurance & to promise that a second bond between mother and daughter is on it's way. In this letter Jessica grants herself permission to feel the heaviness of all of her emotions, whether they be joyful or traumatic.

While awaiting her bundle, she bravely grieves the passing of her first born. A darling baby girl who was born so perfect, yet still. What a privilege to welcome & hold a little angel like she ... what a sensational pink sky she gave this world.

With utter selflessness, these words are written to help any other woman who is pregnant again after going through such crippling loss. For her, for you, from Jessica with weighted love.

Dear me,

There are so many words I have for you as you hold your little bundle of joy, Amélie; crying, staring back at you. Those big blue eyes that you know Evelina would have, but you never got to see sparkle. The soft touch of her hands, the full head of hair and that peaceful demure all mimic Evie's grace and calm. You feel her in the room as you sit wishing she was there, holding her baby sister's hand.

The journey to motherhood for you? Oh, what a journey it has been. The ocean of grief you never thought you would have to travel swallowed you up as you crashed back down under its black billowing waves. Again, and again, and again. While the waves retreat the waters remain eery and when they do arise, they crash and pull you under, leaving you wondering if you will ever take another breath. But you return for air, for there is a new hope. Some lightness. A new life, a sister. With this lightness comes fear, fear of an again. Fear of the unknown. Your innocence has been ripped from beneath your feet while wondering what you did to deserve this everlasting pain. Pain, which you will learn, will never leave you. But in time, you will learn that life and pain coexist. This is terrifying to hear, to feel, to know that it will never go away.

Through this journey of grief and pregnancy after loss you will learn so much about yourself, your friends, and the world that surrounds us.

You will learn to ride the waves knowing that if you fall, you will resurface. Sometimes battered and bruised, sometimes scared, and sometimes ok. You know your husband, your lifeline, will always be standing beside you, holding your hand so tightly you will never drown.

You will learn that your loved ones will do anything for you. They will work night and day to make sure you know they are there. For anything. The love you will feel from them is impenetrable and everlasting. You will feel so incredibly lucky, but so incredibly unlucky at the same time – the purest dichotomy of life.

You will learn that previously considered loved ones will fade away. They want no part in your grief. This will hurt deeply, but in time you will feel grateful that while this pain feels so raw and is a separate loss, you know who is with you for life.

You will learn that people will say the wrong thing. People who are close to you. You are bewildered how they do not realise how deeply upset it makes you. In time this anger will turn to acceptance and the understanding that sometimes some guidance is needed, and that is ok. That they are trying their best. And for those who do not wish to learn, well they will become a part of a life before Evie. This, too, is ok.

You will learn that it's ok to be scared, it's ok to be fearful, it's ok to assume the worst. This is natural, the worst has happened before and it can happen again; there are no guarantees in life. Choose who you share your feelings of deep fear and worry with. Some will show compassion, others may dismiss you with everything will be fine just relax ... stay positive ... don't worry. But how ... you will wonder, how can you say that so confidently? How can you make me feel so unvalidated.

You will make peace that it is ok to take a step back from relationships when you need to.

You will learn that you can love deeply and feel happiness again. These joys will not be stolen from you, though fear will tell you the opposite.

Some weeks will be filled with daily hospital visits, in a state of induced panic. Others will feel oddly calm, like Evie is right there beside you, saying 'it's ok mum, I'm here and I've got you.' You will learn to bask in these moments for while they may be fleeting, they are to be cherished.

You will learn that you can feel so much that it makes you numb. You approach the end like a robot on autopilot. All you need to do is get to 37+1, two days earlier than Evie grew her wings. Such a simple theory to most, but such a minefield for you. You feel blank, and empty. You are scared, so scared. You miss Evie with every ounce of your being. The pain some days is unbearable.

You will learn that a miracle can happen merely 10 months after the most tragic experience of ones life. The moment of Amelie's arrival will be etched in your heart, soul and being, forever. She is here you say, she is here. But Evie, is not. The purest form of happiness and relief, and the deepest of devastation a mother can experience.

As you look into Amelie's big blue eyes, your heart fills with love. Again. You are so proud of your girls. The road ahead is not linear, this much you know. But you will navigate it with your closest few, those who have held your hand and who pull you out from life's quicksand.

You look above your bed each morning at the sunset that sits over you and together you and Amelie say good morning to Evie each day, and goodnight each evening. The strongest bond between sisters that will never be broken, they are tied by the invisible string of love. One which you will bind your family together with forever.

... for little E x

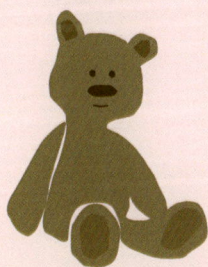

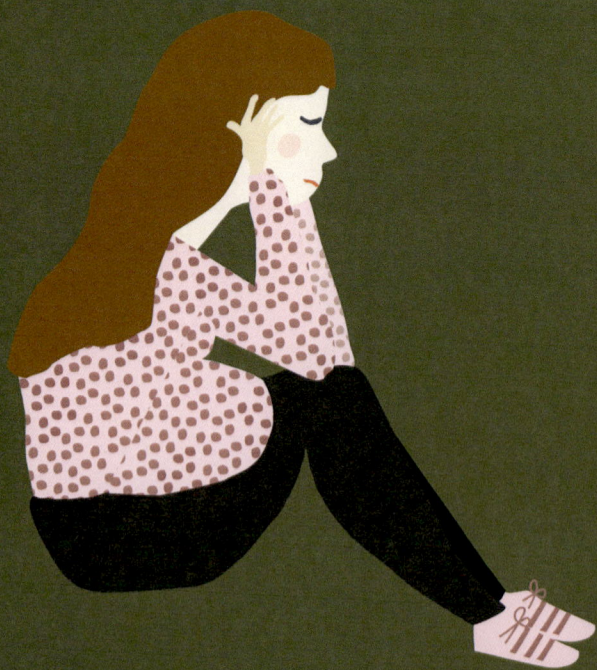

MENTAL HEALTH

... ooft. For some mental health is an issue that doesn't even cross their mind. For others however, the impact pregnancy has on their mental health can feel heavier than the pregnancy itself. Perhaps not for the entirety of it, but certainly during particular stages, which could be weeks, days or just hours. Regardless of their lifespan, the impact is cruel.

The most important thing to establish before we launch into a brilliant chat with a wonderful psychologist who has kindly woven her wisdom into the pages of this book, is that the most positive way to begin confronting darker times is to recognise & admit that you are having a rough time and you need help. Feelings of lethargy, worry, sadness, stress, anxiety or just plain old discomfort in your own skin, mind or home, are not feelings you want to house while growing a baby. The pregnant body has enough to deal with.

We hear so much about postnatal depression – and for good reason – but poor old prenatal depression doesn't tend to get the same air time. Depression, anxiety and a whole other myriad of mental health hiccups can take hold prenatally just as much as they can hit you postnatally.

During my first pregnancy I experienced nothing but feelings of excitement, happiness and a deep maternal yearning. I certainly also had many hormonal dips but for the most part I felt stable.

My second pregnancy however was not as seamless. While I genuinely adore being pregnant, during the first few weeks of round two, I bumped into some of my old mates, aka my depressive triggers. Feelings of numbness and isolation are the stand outs. I tend to drift into an existence of just going through the daily motions like a moving cloud. When I realised I was doing this, from my previous experiences with depression, I knew I'd have to closely monitor myself from then on.

To give you an insight into how this feels I've pasted the original introduction I wrote for the Mental Health chapter of this book, below. Reading back, it's almost a letter to myself. And not an overly colourful or bright one. If this resonates with some readers I hope it enables you to feel as if you are not alone. Because you are far, far from alone.

ON ONE CLOUDY DAY

"I am 5 or 6 weeks pregnant with my second baby and I am feeling so many feelings. Or, to be very honest, I don't think I actually feel much at all? It's hard to differentiate. Who cares.

I'm hosting a level of exhaustion that parallels nothing from my previous pregnancy. I'm just waking up & slipping into an automated set of motions. Wake, exercise, get toddler up, drink coffee, skim the news headlines, shower, eat, work, play, organise, clean, wash, feed, bath, read, pat, sleep. It's just a cycle of movements at the moment. It's not exactly inspiring is it? Hey mojo! Where the f **k are you? I need you.

If you read my first book AFTERWARDS, you'll know that during my first pregnancy I chose to come off my antidepressants, which I take to help a chemical imbalance that's followed me around like a bad smell for years. For the duration of the entire pregnancy, as well as the first 6 months of breastfeeding, I coped swimmingly! Surprising well as I just assumed someone with a predisposition for depression, would struggle with postpartum depression for sure. But I was flourishing in a sunny field of mental wellness I'd never really experienced before. Happiness was **easy**. Innate. All consuming in the best of ways.

Until it wasn't anymore. Like a horrible bad habit, it crawled back into my bones. 'It' being depression. I started to float away into that unpleasant place I dread and dislike. A place I've been so many times before so while it's familiar, it's never comfortable. But with evil ease, it welcomes me back with open arms. I knew at that point, I needed help.

When I came off my medication last time, as I said I felt absolutely fine. I was very much able to cope, I was upbeat and super energised. I was excited and I existed with the most wonderful anticipation. My first baby was on the way! Pop a bottle of non-alcoholic champagne! Grab a mocktail, it's party time!

This time round? Gosh it couldn't be more different.

I've been off the meds for about a week now — a decision I made simply because it's what I did last time. Unlike last time though, I feel like I'm both trying to ground my feet and catch my breath at the same time. I feel flat, low and hidden away from the place I like to hang out — life. I'm tired beyond belief. Unattached, disconnected. I'm worried that I am here again... or there again ... or wherever the hell it is that I am. I need help because unlike last time, I have a toddler to care for now, not to mention a baby growing in my belly. Making my toddler's everyday the best it can be is the reason I get up & chuck on a faux smile. But a faux smile? No thanks, I demand the real deal.

At the moment my ears feel loud. I can hear the workings of my own inner body. Even in the loudest of rooms with ABC Kids blaring and my toddler climbing, chatting, falling, laughing, I can actually hear my skin sitting on my body. I can hear the weight of my bones & the blink of my eyes. It's a chaotic orchestra. It's deafening.

"Do you feel upset or worried about the baby?" — the people close to me ask.

Upset or worried? No, it's not that. It's more like a feeling of spectatorship. I am seeing it all but feeling very little. I am leaning hard into cognitive therapy tactics, as we all tend to do when the lights are dim, & I'm grasping onto things that I recognise and remember make me positive. But it's not working well enough.

Luckily with a toddler in the house, as a mum you're naturally wired to get up & go through the mothering motions without a second thought. You do what you need to do. Feed them, play with them, make them laugh, make them feel protected, warm and loved. Wash them, read to them, rock them, pop them down to sleep. Miss them. Dream of them. Dream with them, for them. They're life's magical little motivators.

Don't get me wrong, I am thrilled to be pregnant!! But with my ol' mate depression re-surfacing, the feelings of connection are beyond my reach. 'Do I return to my meds and introduce a risk (albeit a VERY small risk) to the pregnancy?' This is the question on my mind? And all signs are pointing toward, Yes.

I get quite angry that I can't make my mind just be stronger. 'For godsake, just feel normal Is it really that hard?? The sun is shining, I'm well and healthy and so lucky — what the hell is wrong with me?! Just FEEL BETTER! And then I get frustrated that I'm being so hard on myself. The wonderful empathy of a woman hey? Always on guard, even on the days she is injured.

Depression in all of its various forms, is an illness with its own agenda. It is an illness with its own set of rules, its own schedule, its own motive. Never kind, always hungry.

For anyone else reading this, for anyone who is either pregnant or in the thick of postpartum life, if you share these feelings, I see you.

Anyway I don't have the energy to work towards resolution today. Or keep writing. Tomorrow I'll wake and re-think."

Dark right? Yep. I barely recognise the woman who wrote that. Me.

I never ended up finishing the piece above or writing a 'follow up'. But of course I lived the follow up & it went something like this... I re-read those words and in a heartbeat I made the call to return to antidepressants asap. Why? Because you can only give your family the best version of yourself, when you are the best version. Don't play the martyr mumma. Seek help. It's there.

Moving on to other matters of mental health during pregnancy, as mentioned I was lucky enough to have an open & candid conversation with Elizabeth Neale who has helped me explore a collection of common questions.

DEPRESSION & ANXIETY

Q. Depression as a result of pregnancy, is this common? How do we become aware it & how do we manage it?

Most of us have heard of the Baby Blues, postnatal depression (PND) and postnatal anxiety (PNA), which can all occur after you welcome your baby. As well as this however, around 1 in 10 women in Australia will also experience perinatal depression or perinatal anxiety which presents during the 9 months you're carrying bub. If this is you, don't let it spoil the beauty of your pregnancy as there is help available.

Let's avoid surrounding this topic in too many numbers or statistics as we are all far more than a number on a page. Just because these conditions may be "common," this fact doesn't make it easier for the individual going through it.

Depression general, but especially during pregnancy, can be caused by many reasons. Two of which might be (A) a neurochemical imbalance i.e. what I personally experience or (B) something within your environment has triggered you. For example a previous loss, an unhappy relationship or financial strain. Whatever the cause, whoever falls into this puddle will know that the splash is cold & grim.

Firstly, to differentiate between perinatal depression and perinatal anxiety. The depression side of things is usually when you feel flat, disconnected, noticeably lethargic and/or hopeless. The anxiety side of things on the other hand, is where you may worry, or feel restless, panicked or you'll fear the worst. In other words you'll catastrophize an outcome before it actually happens.

If this sounds familiar, don't panic as you will be ok. With support & appropriate coping mechanisms, you'll get through it.

STEPS TO RECOVER

1. **Visit your GP.** Explain exactly how you're feeling. If you find this too difficult, write it down on paper before your appointment. It doesn't have to be an essay – it could just be a list of emotions or reasons for being there. For example:

   'My name is Tori, I am 32 years old and 27 weeks pregnant. For the past week I've been feeling sad, worried and unable to focus. I've never felt this way. I am in a safe and healthy relationship, with plenty of family support & a job I enjoy. But for some reason I feel down. Can you help?" Or;

   'I'm here because ever since I fell pregnant I haven't felt ok. I cry for no reason. I panic that I'll lose the baby."

2. **Tell your partner or someone close.** Do this either before or after your GP visit. No matter how strong you think you may be, pregnancy is an extremely unprecedented time. Unlike other life experiences, the surge of hormones, the control you lose & the physicality required to grow a baby, will challenge you in new ways.

3. **Seek Light.** On the days or during the moments you feel the worst, find activities (or people), that bring a feeling of lightness or reprieve. Try to distract your mind however possible. From personal experience, I turn to exercise to unleash the smiling rush of endorphins.

   Going for a walk with uplifting music or a podcast (keep the content light folks). Cooking. Reading. Clearing out your wardrobe. Cleaning, (vacuuming is my personal version of meditation), or simply laying on the couch and trying to have a nap. Whatever it takes to lighten or redirect your mind – do it.

4. **Wrap yourself in restful empathy.** When you're clouded by fog, avoid anything or anyone you may find triggering or mentally tiring. An example of this might be social events. It is ok to say no to social invitations! In many situations, it's probably BEST to say no & use the time to rest.

5. **Watch your coffee intake.** Caffeine is a psychostimulant that affects the central nervous system in the brain. Caffeine works by blocking a chemical in our cells called adenosine which is believed to be responsible for increasing the level of 'sleepiness' we feel, hence why coffee heightens our 'awake-ness'.

   When we drink coffee, this chemical process may lead an already anxious person to struggle with feelings of nervousness & restlessness. It can lead to headaches, shakiness or irritability. Give the latte a miss until you're feeling calmer.

6. **Allow time and patience to work through management tools with your GP or Health Care Provider.** Whether you've been advised to talk to someone such as a psychologist, trial medication and/or change certain lifestyle habits, don't expect a cure overnight. Give it time, proactive patience and above all else, give it a chance.

7. **Be Upfront.** Tell your midwife or OBGYN what you're going through & if you've been recommended particular management tools (e.g. physical exercise) or prescribed medication. To provide the safest of care for you, they need all information. No one is going to judge you for looking after yourself!

Above all else – be kind to yourself. Eat good food, rest & spend time with those who make you feel good.

Let's go back a step. How will you know if you're experiencing perinatal depression & not just a shitty mood? The common signs to look out for include:

* A consistently flat mood. For those who are unsure of the term "flat mood," in my experience a flat mood is when you're unable to feel 'varied moods'. You don't feel happy or sad or angry or stressed or excited. You just feel numb & disconnected.
* You experience feelings of worthlessness.
* Your sleeping habits become disturbed.
* There are noticeable changes to your appetite.

* You find yourself crying often over things that wouldn't usually bother you.
* You're feeling unwilling to get up in the morning and unable to cope.
* You're uninterested & dissociated with things & people.
* You experience intense or random bouts of irritability or rage.
* You have suicidal thoughts or thoughts of self-harming.

If you relate to any of the above, it's time to seek help. Make a GP appointment now.

Some women may feel more comfortable inviting a support person (for example your partner) along to the to the appointment, which is totally fine! Great in fact.

For any women however who are reading this & in a position where they feel they can't go alone or they can't tell their partner they're off to a personal appointment – please don't let that stop you. If a sense of control or fear exists within your relationship, or worst yet abuse (whether it be control or physical), you need to call White Ribbon Australia on 1800 RESPECT (i.e. 1800 737 732), and seek support. You can even go onto the White Ribbon Australia website and use their Online Chat function if this option is safer. If required, delete your browsing history.

To close the chapter on mental health, the take home really should be; speak openly with your GP at all times, as well as your midwife, OB, your partner, friends, family or your Doula. Be honest about your feelings and lean into the support & help that will be offered. There is always help available.

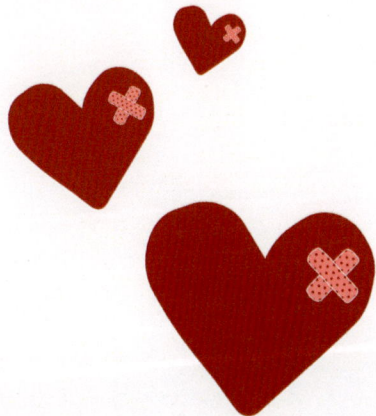

PERINATAL ANXIETY

Q. **Moving onto perinatal anxiety. Is this common? How do we become aware of it & how do we manage it?**

Let's focus solely on anxiety for a moment. Anxiety is a prick isn't it?

While I joke, I don't want to downplay the awful nature of anxiety as it can be crippling. For me, out of depression & anxiety, anxiety is the toughest to manage as it takes complete ownership of my body & mind. It makes me feel like I've had 4 coffees and 3 cans of Red Bull, leaving me to operate in fast forward mode. It's unsustainable & it's yuck.

Anxiety is an emotion or a cluster of emotions that can typically include feelings of worry, nervousness, guilt, tension or 'irrational' fear. During anxious episodes, your blood pressure may increase or you can feel light headed or even 'tipsy'. You may feel on edge or just completely uncomfortable in your own skin. In these moments, if it's available to you, move yourself into a new environment. If you're at work, take yourself outside for 5-10 minutes and focus on slow, deep breathing.

For those suspicious of the effectiveness of deep breathing, let's take a moment here to explore Deep Breathing. Does it work or is it all just codswallop? Yes. It absolutely **does** work. It alters the way our brain and therefore our body performs and behaves.

When we are stressed or anxious we tend to take short, shallow breaths as the body enters it's fight-or-flight mode. Fight-or-flight mode is the body's natural defence mechanism. It kickstarts when it senses an 'attack' coming. The short breath is the body's attempt to get more oxygen to the muscles in preparation to "fight" off the incoming attack.

The problem? This style of quick breathing, commonly referred to as hyperventilation, throws off the balance of gas in our body. A pickle.

The art of breathing is all about absorbing oxygen (on the inhale) and expelling carbon dioxide (on the exhale), through movement of the lungs using our diaphragm. In stressful moments when our breath shortens, our heart rate also tends to rise. This combination can lead us into a hot sweat – exacerbating feelings of panic or anxiety.

By consciously slowing & deepening our breath, we can induce a positive effect. Continuous slow, deep breaths will work to realign the synchronicity between breath & heart rate – which can then encourage the brain to release endorphins, a chemical that has a calming effect. So! While deep breathing won't cure the cause of anxiety, it can manage the symptoms in the moment.

I read a Harvard Business Review from 2020, while preparing to write this chapter. The crux of the Review, summarised below, personally helped me to conceptualise the process of deep breathing. In other words, it helped me understand how to actually do it. There is quite an art to breathing, believe it or not.

'When you inhale, your heart rate speeds up. When you exhale, it slows down. Breathing in for a count of 4 and out for a count of 8 for just a few minutes can start to calm your nervous system. Remember: when you feel agitated, lengthen your exhales.'

From my own experience, anxiety usually presents as an inability to control rational or 'chronological' dialogue in my mind. My thoughts start at A, they go to B, and then back to A, to M, to Y to C, only to end up at the worst case scenario... Z. It's here at Z where I usually fall into a heap, exhausted by the internal war of words. In short, I catastrophize outcomes in my head. Sounds exhausting right? It is.

Speaking to Elizabeth Neale, with her rich and refined perspective, I'm now enlightened with a new understanding of anxiety during pregnancy. Elizabeth posed this question to me. 'Can palatable amounts of these anxious feelings be used as a helpful tool?" *Keep in mind that we're strictly isolating this question around the topic of pregnancy.* So can they? Can small amounts of worry or panic be used to **help** us **prepare** and **cope** when heading into the unknown i.e. life with a baby?

OR, what about looking at it this way; can we turn negative thoughts and assumptions during this time into positive emotions with added value? In short, yes. We are capable of doing this.

Before continuing, I must reiterate that some women reading this **will** need more substantial help from a professional in this field (such as Elizabeth Neale), and/or medication to deal with more debilitating bouts of anxiety. While a certain amount of Cognitive Behaviour Therapy (CBT) (a type of therapy that involves challenging our personal patterns of behaviour by using problem solving techniques to adapt our way of thinking) can help some people, others will need a stronger remedy.

Don't be upset if this is you. It's been me before & I promise the light at the end of the tunnel will rear its head soon.

Where was I? … oh yes! For those who are struggling with a level of anxiety that we can try and manage using CBT, can we turn anxiety into a valuable tool? Or a preparation tool? We can try!

When we predict an upsetting outcome, what can you do now to prevent the upsetting outcome from eventuating? Can you change upcoming plans? Can you make particular arrangements? Can you strengthen your knowledge about whatever it is you're fearful of? Can you seek help and find ways to cope if what you were worried about did eventuate?

Can you break a situation down, turn it into a list and tick off the elements one-by-one. This way, instead of one big and stressful task, it becomes bite sized, do-able tasks. The feeling of gratification along the way can be hugely beneficial to your mental health.

In short mummas-to-be, when it comes to protecting your mental health, it's about finding ways to manage. If you fear your baby is not going to sleep, start doing some light reading or chat to friends about their experiences. There is merit in the old saying 'prepare for the worst & expect the best." The key word being – prepare.

WARNING: if, however a feeling of shame creeps into your anxious episodes, monitor this closely as shame is the most toxic element of anxiety. Shame can be defined a 'as painful feeling of humiliation or distress caused by the consciousness of wrong or foolish behaviour'. Shame is a feeling that can quickly erode your self-worth and cripple your ability to think straight and feel adequate. If you feel a sense of shame about yourself, please seek help immediately. The below sources are a great place to start:

* Your local GP
* Your partner, a trusted friend or family member
* Beyond Blue Healthy Families healthyfamilies.org.au
* PANDA www.panda.org.au

BODY IMAGE

Q. Let's look at body disorder issues as a result of pregnancy. The relationship between a woman and her body can be a very complicated one, we all know that. If a woman is struggling to identify herself or feel content in her own skin during pregnancy, are there ways to rationalise these feelings?

This is when you have to dig deep and harness your most rational self. Elizabeth, our wonderful psychologist, considers the matter in a succinct and very reasonable way.

To have a baby, there are 'certain things' that *must* happen. The word *must* is the crucial element of this topic. For example, one thing that *must* happen to have a baby, is your body has to change.

Without particular changes to our bodies during pregnancy, the dream, to birth a child, is not possible. It's as simple as that really isn't it? Think of it this way;

* Your own body will grow as another human body (or multiple), grows inside you.
* Your weight will increase as the baby grows.
* Not only does the actual baby add kilos but you'll also have an increased blood supply, more fluid, a placenta, a heavier uterus muscle and potentially bigger boobs. It all adds up.
* Being pregnant means your hips are likely to widen as your body naturally prepares for a safe and comfortable delivery. In order to minimise injury & prevent damage, your hips widening is a very, very good thing.
* As we touched on, your boobs are likely to grow as the level of estrogen and progesterone increase as the pregnancy advances. These hormones prepare your boobs for lactation. Milk!
* Your appetite is likely to change or increase. Maybe not everyday, but certainly on some. Why? Just like going for a big run, your body is using a lot of energy to grow your baby, every single minute of the day. The increased energy used is what can cause your hunger levels to change. On this note, just remember that eating does not always translate to weight gain. Eating translates to nourishing your unborn baby. Oh, and surviving.

In short; You are not fat. You are pregnant! But it's OK and NORMAL to have days where you feel a little down about the changes your body is undergoing. Of courseeeee it is!!!

Self Admission! Just because I'm sounding so matter-of-fact here, it does not mean that I'm immune to body image issues during pregnancy. Hell no! During the first trimester of my 2nd pregnancy, I'd go into the chemist to weigh myself. You know what happened? The number on the scales WENT UP! Every single bloody time! You know why?! Because I was pregnant! And *thankfully* my baby was growing!

I swear that before they are our babies, they are our muffin tops!

Even though the subject of body image during pregnancy may seem superficial when compared to other subjects such as fertility & birth – if you do suffer from body image issues, it is absolutely a subject of value which requires support.

Elizabeth suggested that if you align your worth and self-esteem primarily with your appearance, the danger can be the daily attack on your self-identity. To correct this, we have to change our perspective. Like this:

INSTEAD OF...	TRY...
I am fat.	No, I am pregnant.
My ankles are so chubby.	No, my ankles are carrying more fluid due to the pregnancy. The fluid will subside after the birth.
The size of my hips is disgusting.	No, my hips are widening so I can safely deliver the baby. I am lucky.

Justify the self deprecation with the matter-of-fact.

If you have previously suffered from body issues or disordered eating prior to falling pregnant, this road is likely to be more challenging for you. Seeking support from a trusted health care provider is a good idea. If this is you, rest assured you're not alone.

Discussing ways to shield any triggers with your GP or midwife is a very good idea. For example, if you would prefer not to know your weight as the weeks go on, ask that they monitor the scales & make notes without you seeing. And pleaseeee don't be embarrassed to do this! Otherwise look to the many wonderful organisations for support around the clock. These two are great starters;

* Eating Disorders Org – www.eatingdisorders.org.au
* Butterfly Foundation – www.butterfly.org.au/get-support/helpline

If you do have a history with disordered eating or if you're all of a sudden struggling with it during your pregnancy, tell your midwife, your OB and/or your GP so they can provide the very best & most relevant care for you. If you keep it to yourself & let the issue escalate, the risks *can* be damaging for both you & baby.

Please Note: The word *can* is emphasised above as this chapter is not meant to evoke fear or panic. It is intended to highlight why seeking support is so important.

* Intra-uterine Growth Restriction
* Miscarriage
* Labor Complications
* Pre-term Birth (when the baby is born before they are fully developed)
* The baby having a low birth weight
* If you have an eating disorder, you may also be at higher risk of experiencing postnatal depression (PND).

MEDICATION DURING PREGNANCY

Q. **If I take prescribed medication for a mental health issue, should I keep taking it or come off it during pregnancy?**

Elizabeth notes that this is a very personal matter and one that absolutely requires medical advice, knowledge and counsel from your GP.

For those interested, my story is below but please do not base your own decisions around mine. Everyone's heath, pregnancy & circumstances are wildly varied.

I came off my anti-depressants during my first pregnancy as, given it was my first pregnancy, nearly every possible risk worried me. I chose to eliminate 'potential' risks, regardless of how small they were considered. If I felt OK without them, I'd continue … if not, I would go back to my doctor & reconsider. To my genuine surprise, I felt fine. Better actually! As the weeks & months flew by, I absolutely loved pregnancy life. The happiness I felt batted away any & all triggers. Thinking back on it, I STILL feel warm and fuzzy about that time in my life.

Post birth however & around 6 months into breastfeeding, I felt the old triggers nudge their way back. I felt low, distracted and disconnected. No thanks. After talking to my GP, I chose to return to my meds. After doing so, the fog took about a week or so to fade. I had a period of locked jaw, restlessness and a funny tummy but all of that was a small price to pay to get my life back on track. Hello world!

My second pregnancy was different. After talking to my GP I once again chose to come off the meds. But just 5 or 6 days later I knew it was a poor choice. I felt hellish. Foggy, low, distracted with terrible OCD tendencies (such as having to touch something 'x' number of times ... placing household items in a particular order before I let myself go on with the day ... clicking my tongue ... subconsciously reciting little mantras in my head... f**k it's exhausting). With a toddler in tow, I had zero patience for feeling like crap.

Back to the GP I went. I was desperate to hear her clinical advice and get her 'approval' to return to medication. Instead I received a series of wise words, which I still cherish. '*A pregnant woman who is mentally fit, able to cope and energised – is a healthy pregnant woman & a strong person. For your baby to be OK, you need to be OK.*'

That was all it took. Meds hello & once again, hello world! I won't sugar-coat this decision too much as I carried a lot of guilt over the nine months (and still to this day as I breastfeed). Why the guilt? There are always potential risks when medication is introduced into the human body (pregnant or not). Guilt is another bitch of a feeling – but one that can be rationalised in this instance. For my baby to be OK, I need to be OK.

If you suffer from a mental illness, you deserve to accept the help that is available to you – and without shame.

When making decisions such as these, Elizabeth encourages the need to be completely honest with yourself. The checklist below may help, but the first port of call should always be your GP.

* Am I getting through the day?
* Am I able to cope with the daily tasks?
* Do I feel lethargic & distracted by the fog that surrounds me?
* Am I able to hold my focus?
* Do I feel safe?
* Do I feel confident about this pregnancy?

Regardless of how many Yes VS No's you get – see your GP.

SELF DOUBT

Q. **The fears around not wanting the baby once it arrives or not being a capable mother.... When self doubt is deafening, how can women overcome it?**

I think we all bump into these worries don't we? I used to worry that I wouldn't like spending so much time with a baby. I feared I'd be bored, restless and resentful. I would think back to my babysitting days and remember the stench of old milk & the freedom I embraced with SO much excitement when the parents arrived home & let me escape.

Women fear they won't love or connect with their baby. They fear they'll blame their baby for robbing them of their time and their old life. Women fear they won't know how to properly feed and nourish their baby adequately. Women are haunted with fears of miscarriage, stillbirth, complications during labor and/or emergency situations unravelling during or post delivery. Women fear their babies won't love them.

We ALL fear something. Hell, I feared the cooking aspect of motherhood to the tenth degree! Post breastfeeding, will this baby also like to eat tuna, salmon, packet rice or salad?! Probably NOT! Even the thought of getting my child fed everyday (let alone 3 or more times per day), riddled me with fear & self doubt. To be honest, my eldest is now 3 and it STILL does.

Silly? Sure! But the fear is real.

On a more serious level, I feared the loss of my time & my identity. The loss of my freedom to work and live independently. Unlike the cooking fear, this one actually kept me up for hours at night during my first pregnancy. But I say this to you *without a word of a lie*, if you cherish something within your life outside motherhood (in my case, my career), you will *always* make it work. You are capable of much more than you think mumma, trust me.

If self doubt takes you into deep & dark territory however, for example if you fear you will not want your baby post birth, please give yourself the benefit of the doubt and speak to your GP for added guidance. Like we touched on earlier in this chapter ... if you can work out ways to manage particular situations & occurrences should they arise, *before* they arise, you will feel stronger and more confident in your ability to cope.

Worrying is perhaps inevitable for many of us. Those sleepless hours between 1am and 4am are heinous, yet all too familiar. For now, take a deep breath and try to think forward to positive moments. Inside, you're holding a little person who, if you allow them to , will reflect the best parts of you. Inside you is a heart that will naturally connect with yours because you are family. You will be a beautiful mother. Your child will love their wonderful mum.

To close the chapter on mental health, the take home really should be; speak openly with your GP at all times, as well as your midwife, OB, your partner, friends, family or your Doula. Be honest about your feelings and lean into the support & help that will be offered. There is always help available.

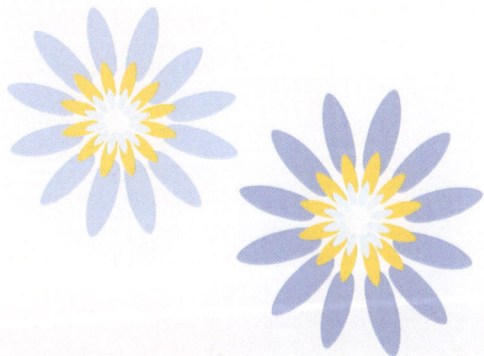

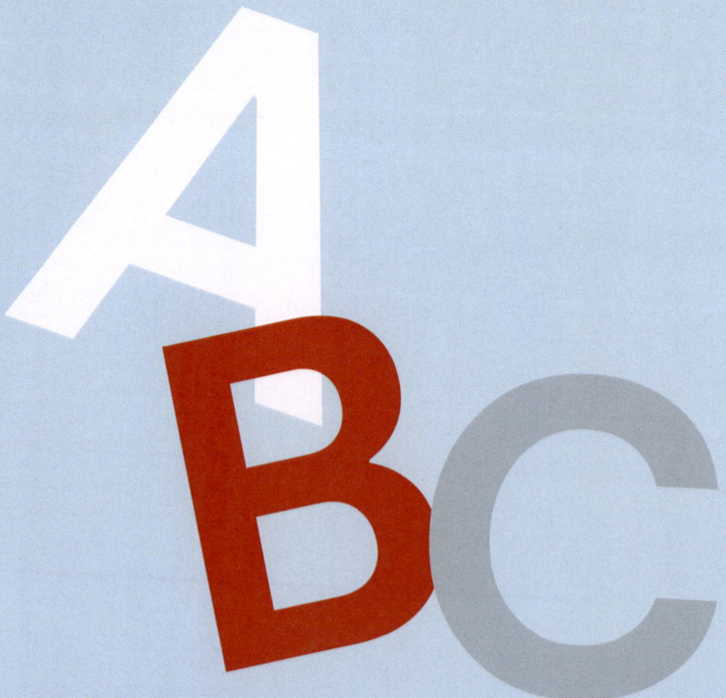
ABC

COMMON BIRTH TERMS

Heading into hospital for the birth was always something I was afraid of while pregnant. For some reason, the clinical nature of hospitals scare me a little. Machines flash & beep. The corridors are lined with gurneys & wheelchairs. The fluorescent lighting is stark & bright. The general atmosphere is a little sterile for someone who is not used to this type of enviroment. The maternity ward however should be thought of as a happy place. A safe, comfortable & exciting space where babies enter the world!

The good news is that the people who work in the maternity wards, are magic. The midwives and nurses are wonderfully kind. They glow with joy & empathy and they fill the ward with bubbly anticipation. And they just LOVE babies & they LOVE delivering babies!

I personally love them because they have access to the drugs ... i.e. the pain medication that can help women get through the gruelling marathon that is labor. What is not to love about that? Of course there are women who prefer labor without drugs, and this is amazing too! In fact I salute you. To me, you're bloody superhuman.

Feeling comfortable in a hospital & on the maternity ward in particular, may feel far less daunting if you do some homework now and learn about some common birthing lingo, to lessen the number of surprises on the day.

I am so fortunate to welcome Tahlia O'Rourke into these pages, to help guide us through the birthing glossary. Tahlia founded Wolfe&Cub in 2020 – the home to a range of both private & group workshops – that cover everything within the prenatal & postnatal realm.

Tahlia is a passionate midwife, a registered nurse and a mother to her darling baby. She is a walking body of knowledge, so thank goodness we've hijacked her bustling mind to explain the MANY terms we are likely to hear over the course of pregnancy, birth & postpartum. Like myself, Tahlia would like to caution that nothing below is to be taken as medical advice or strict direction. Anything & everything to do with your health, your pregnancy, your baby & your birth should always be checked by your personal GP, midwife or OB.

For more of her guidance & expertise, find Tahlia @wolfe.and.cub
Or do yourself a favour & book in a workshop!

In alphabetical order, below are a few very common 'terms', that may help ease any curiosities prior to birth!

B IS FOR
BREECH BABY

A Breech baby is a baby who is bottom down or feet first in your uterus. It's likely that at more than one point during your pregnancy, your baby may be in that position. They are like little acrobats in the womb, constantly on the move! Especially early in your pregnancy. Breech babies are more likely during a woman's first pregnancy when the muscles of the uterus are nice and relaxed. Breech babies are more likely if this is not your first baby and the muscles of your uterus are nice and relaxed, previous breech baby, a low-lying placenta, too much or too little fluid around your baby, an uncommon uterus shape fibroids or a multiple pregnancy.

As you reach the final months of your pregnancy, you'll notice that your care provider will place more emphasis on the position of your baby and will likely address it with you more often. A breech vaginal birth may be achievable if your birthing facility can facilitate that (if it's safe & suitable for you of course). They'll take into consideration many elements, including the type of breech baby you have on board, and of course your desire to make that happen. Your body, your baby.

If your baby is still breech around the 36 week mark, it's unlikely that your baby will turn to head down by itself (unlikely, but not impossible). You may be offered what is called an External Cephalic Version (ECV). An ECV can be performed by a qualified member of the obstetric team. The procedure involves manually turning your baby from a bottom down position to a head first position by placing gentle pressure on your abdomen with their hands. The aim is to guide your baby to do a somersault. As you can imagine the procedure often involves a level of uncomfortableness. Medication can be given to help relax your uterus to aid in the turning of your baby. There is a 50/50 chance that this procedure will be successful. There are certain criteria that need to be met for an ECV to be performed. This discussion will be had with your birthing team.

If your baby is breech and you don't like the sound of an ECV, you may like to try different positional exercises, acupuncture, a visit to a chiropractor or moxibustion (moxibustion is an of external treatment based on the theory of traditional Chinese medicine). Of course it's always recommended of course medical advice before trying anything new or booking yourself into any appointment for an intervention.

If the bub doesn't turn on their own, it's likely you will be offered an elective caesarean birth. With all of this in mind it is so important that you feel comforted, educated & empowered in your decision making. Cheeky, challenging little babies.

E IS FOR
EPIDURAL

An epidural is a medical form of pain relief that helps a mother feel an altered sensation and numbness from the top of the uterus down to her toes, in turn contributing to a pain free labor.

An anaesthetist performs the epidural procedure. There are a few things that need to happen first to make an epidural possible.

Firstly, a cannula will need to be inserted to enable the administration of fluids, to make sure that both you & your baby are well hydrated prior to the procedure.

A blood test will be performed to assess your suitability for the procedure. The anaesthetist will then talk you through the procedure and gain your consent prior to moving forward.

Next, both the midwife caring for you and the anaesthetist will work on positioning you to enable the procedure to be performed. It's likely that you will be sitting on the side of the bed, hunched forward with your back towards the anaesthetist. Keep in mind there can be a lot of repositioning involved to make sure you are in the ideal position for the procedure. Try and relax. Deep breaths.

Your back will then be thoroughly cleaned with an antiseptic solution and a plastic drape will be popped over you to maintain a sterile field, decreasing the risk of infection associated with the procedure. Once the sterile drape is placed over your back it's hugely important that your support person doesn't touch your back at any point (e.g. by trying to comfort you), as this will impact sterility & the process will need to be redone.

The anaesthetist will now administer local anaesthetic which numbs the skin on your back. You may feel a slight sting ... or even the flush of a bee sting sensation. The administering of the local anaesthetic ensures the rest of the procedure is as painless as possible.

Staying as still as possible is now the goal. Keeping in mind that stillness can be very difficult when you're experiencing painful contractions, you'll be encouraged to focus on your breathing & asked to communicate any needs to your support person or midwife, to ensure you don't move.

A needle is then gently guided into your back between the bones of your spine, into what is called the epidural space. Once it's in the correct place, the needle is then removed leaving a small plastic tube in your back. The plastic tube is the source of the pain relief medication which will be administered throughout your labor and birth. It'll be secured by tape to your back, so you won't have to worry about it moving.

An epidural will remain in place until you have brought your baby earthside. Following this (the main event!), the epidural will be turned off, allowing your body to regain sensation in the hours that follow. When you're given the all clear, you'll be able to move freely.

It is worth noting [that unless your birthing facility uses a walking epidural] after the epidural has been administered, your movement becomes very restricted (it's unsafe to attempt walking or standing when you lack feeling in your legs).

From this point you're likely to remain in the bed for the labor and birth of your baby. Your baby will require continuous heart rate monitoring. A catheter will be inserted into you to drain urine from your bladder as you'll be unable to walk to the bathroom. The catheter is commonly removed within 24 hours of birthing your baby. However this is dependant on your own individual

F IS FOR
FORCEPS

Forceps are smooth, spoon-shaped instruments that hold, support and protect your baby's head as a member of the obstetric team gently pulls to help assist your baby through the birth canal & out of the vagina, bringing them earthside in the safest possible way. They are not required in all deliveries.

H IS FOR
HIGH BLOOD PRESSURE

Blood Pressure is a recording of the pressure pushing against your blood vessel walls as your heart beats.

Your blood pressure in pregnancy and throughout your life is an indication of the overall health of your heart and blood vessels.

So why is blood pressure monitoring important in pregnancy? Adequate pumping of blood and oxygen around your body results in the overall health and wellbeing of your growing baby. If you have high blood pressure it is possible that your baby may not be receiving as much nourishment compared to a baby who's mum has normal blood pressure. The reason being, the nutrients travelling to your baby via the placenta, could be restricted. If this occurs it can affect the overall growth of your baby & in more severe cases, it can lead to further pregnancy complications such as premature birth, placental abruption and pre-eclampsia.

Some women need their blood pressure to be monitored more regularly throughout their pregnancy and in some cases may be started on medication.

I IS FOR
INDUCTION

From time to time it may be recommended to help bring your baby earth-side prior to going into labor on your own. This proposal can often be associated with feelings of fear & even disappointment. Midwives get it & are there to help you understand what is involved & to encourage you to make it your own.

Examples of times where an IOL (Induction Of Labor) may be offered include:

* A pregnancy of 41 weeks onwards
* Your waters have broken & your labor has not begun after some time
* Concerns for your bubs movements, growth or amniotic fluid
* Gestational Diabetes
* High blood pressure

Methods of IOL do differ from mum to mum, hospital to hospital, however it may happen as follows:

* Firstly, the ripening of your cervix with prostaglandin hormone in the form of gel (Prostin) or tape (Cervidil) inserted into the vagina. A midwife or OB can perform this with your consent. It is our hope for you that this medication works it's magic helping to shorten & soften the cervix getting you ready for your labor.
* Another method that may be used is called a cooks catheter. For the placement you may be asked to put your legs in stirrups. The vagina is then opened with a speculum (much like a pap smear) then the catheter,

a thin plastic tube is positioned into the cervix. Once in, a small balloon is inflated inside & outside the cervical opening to place pressure on the cervix resulting in dilation & falling out of the balloon. This will indicate your body's readiness to progress in labor.

* Once your cervix is open 1-2cm a Midwife or OB will break your waters by performing an artificial rupture of membranes (ARM)

* Sometimes the hormonal shift in your waters breaking can start labor alone however, if this does not happen for you, the love hormone oxytocin, will be offered to you via a drip in its medical form, Syntocinon which will assist in creating strong, regular contractions bringing you closer to the birth of your baby. Slow & steady, the drip will then be increased to assist in the progression of your labor.

* Throughout an IOL, your bubs heart rate will be monitored using continuous monitoring (CTG)

You've got this!

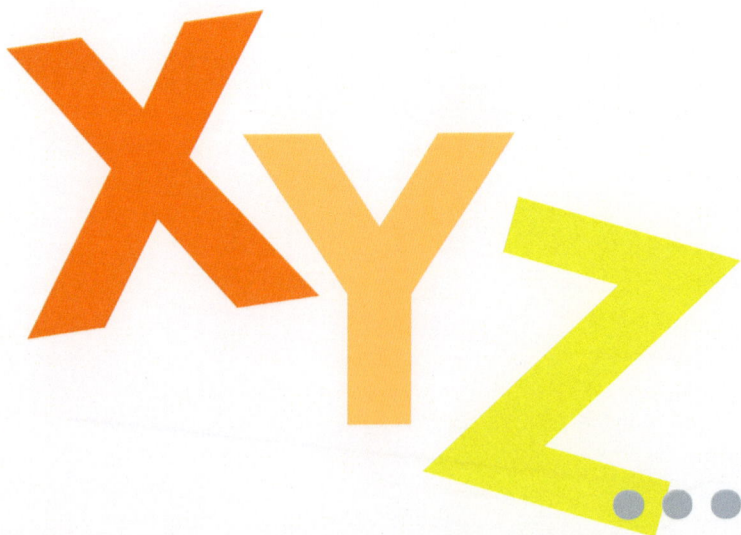

V IS FOR
VACUUM

A vacuum, also known as a ventouse, is a soft flat cup that is inserted and placed on top of your baby's head. A member of the obstetric team will then use a hand held pump, attached to the cup, resulting in suction (much like a plunger) to enable them to gently pull to help assist your baby through the birth canal & out of the vagina, bringing them earthside in the safest possible way.

For both assisted delivery methods (i.e. Forceps or the use of the Vacuum), it is worth noting:

An assisted delivery requires a calm environment, good & clear communication between the health care professional & the mother & of course, consent to the procedure.

With contractions, the team caring for you will encourage you to push as the Doctor gently pulls. There is no pulling without pushing. In many cases it's likely you will require an episiotomy to assist in the birth of your baby. This can create more space for the use of instruments, it can decrease the likelihood of sustaining a vaginal tear & it may also decrease the amount of pressure placed higher up within the birth space i.e. your pelvic floor muscles.

The decision to use instruments for the assisted birth of your baby is driven by the need for safety, of the mother or the baby. If safety is jeopardised by time – waiting for normal birth to occur – it may be necessary for the birthing team to use interventions to hurry the birth process along.

PRE-ECLAMPSIA

Hands up who experienced this... ME!! I had pre-eclampsia with my little boy. Pre-eclampsia is high blood pressure and more. It involves multiple organs and not only does it affect your blood pressure reading, but it can also affect certain levels in your urine and blood. In its most serious form, pre-eclampsia can lead to seizures, stroke, bleeding, placental abruption, organ failure, abnormal growth of your baby and premature birth.

Some common signs and symptoms include, but are not limited to: headaches, visual disturbances (like seeing stars/blurry vision), swelling particularly in the hands, face and feet (ankles... what are ankles), pain particularly below the ribs and generally just feeling unwell.

Once you have a diagnosis of pre-eclampsia, it's not until your baby is born that it subsides. In some cases it may actually continue into the postnatal period. Pre-eclampsia can be a reason to induce labor or opt for a caesarean birth, as both can assist in the safety & wellbeing of the mother and the baby.

It's important that your blood pressure continues to be monitored, medication considered and weaning commences as well as a thorough 6 week check (to include blood pressure monitoring), to ensure all is well post birth . Your hospital stay may be prolonged to ensure your blood pressure is stable prior to discharge home with your new baby.

If you want more information regarding these terms & their explanations, please talk to your health care provider. Knowledge is power mumma!

Grief Tips – Post Stillbirth and Loss

The list of suggestions below is written by Jessica, for anyone who may know someone who has tragically lost a baby.

1. Check in a lot for the first 2 or 3 months after. Daily if your friend is responsive to it. Let them know you are there. Equally, if they ask for space please respect it.

2. Asking simply questions such as, 'How are you?' is very important … rather than saying 'I hope you are well," or "I hope you are ok'. Asking, 'How are you?' signifies that you are ok with any answer, whether its dark / light / sad or devastating. Saying 'I hope you are well' to someone grieving, can come across like you don't want to know or you'd prefer not to deal with the answer.

3. Mention your friends babies name a LOT. As a loss mum you feel like a childless mum & you feel as though your baby is going to be forgotten. Or worse, never existed as people don't talk about them. There is nothing more heartwarming than knowing your baby is on your friends mind.

4. Avoid asking – What do you need? … or Let me know if you need anything? They can barely get out of bed let alone work out what they need. Waking up in those first few months is the worst part of the day because you realise you're still alive and baby is not. Just sent texts, food, a random gift or acknowledge what they're going through. For some, phone calls will feel impossible, so instead it's so lovely receiving something thoughtful out of the blue … even just a text.

5. Just listen. That's all we need. There are no answers when you loose a child. There is no "at least this…" or "at least that…', or "you'll have another baby." Let us grieve. We don't need a solution. All we need is a hug and to know that you're not going to disappear.

6. You can't 'fix' them, so please don't try. They will never be 'healed' or find peace with the fact their baby died. Time does not heal this wound. Instead we just have to learn to live alongside the pain.

7. Chat to them normally when the time is right, as in, how you used to. They are still them, they are just going through something incredibly difficult. In those early days I used to love when my friends would tell me to watch a random show, send me a silly meme or just say something detached from what I was going through. It lightened my brain for a minute, and that was so welcomed.

8. Ask them if they'd like to be included in things (social things), but don't make them feel pressured to say yes. 'Hi, I'm going for a walk this morning at 10 if you'd like to join?' Leave the ball in their court. This way, they won't feel pressured & they won't feel as though they're letting you down if they are unable to make it.

9. They will sweat the small stuff. Just expect it. Everything is magnified right now. They feel like they should have this grand & brand new perspective, but that will take time to come (if at all). If they are behaving irrationally about things they wouldn't usually care about, please remember this will pass. Their brain is in a chaotic washing machine right now. They will get there! It's just a process.

10. Ask them how they are feeling physically. Everyone forgets about this. They still gave birth to a baby and they were pregnant for however many months. Night sweats, dealing with milk coming in, uterus contractions, tears, C-Sections. We go through all of this too. The difference is, we recover without our baby.

11. If you are close enough with them, ask if they need help with any administrative tasks. I will never forget when

my bestfriend asked me if I needed help with the admin processes while I was planning our baby's cremation & an urn for her ashes. While I didn't accept her offer it meant the world to me and I will honestly never forget that level of care. There are hospital forms, Centrelink forms, Medicare, funeral arrangements, cremation, organisation of the certificate of birth and death. The list is endless and it feels so overwhelming at the time!

12. Put their babies monthly birth date in your diary and text every month for the first 6 months. It means so much. Just a little, 'Thinking of you and your baby (name) today. They are so loved and you are so loved.'

13. Christmas, Easter, Holidays and Birthdays for the first year are awful. Send a little text saying, 'I'm sorry today sucks and it wasn't meant to be like this. I love you.' A simple text like this is literally all they may need sometimes. It means so much.

14. Try to avoid telling them they're strong. When you loose a child, you feel like you have no alternate option than to keep living. This is not 'being strong', this is surviving. Being told they're 'strong' makes them feel as if they have to act strong, and that they can't let their walls down.

15. Remember that everyone is learning and nobody is perfect. Your friend will be so appreciative if you read resources such as these to offer support.

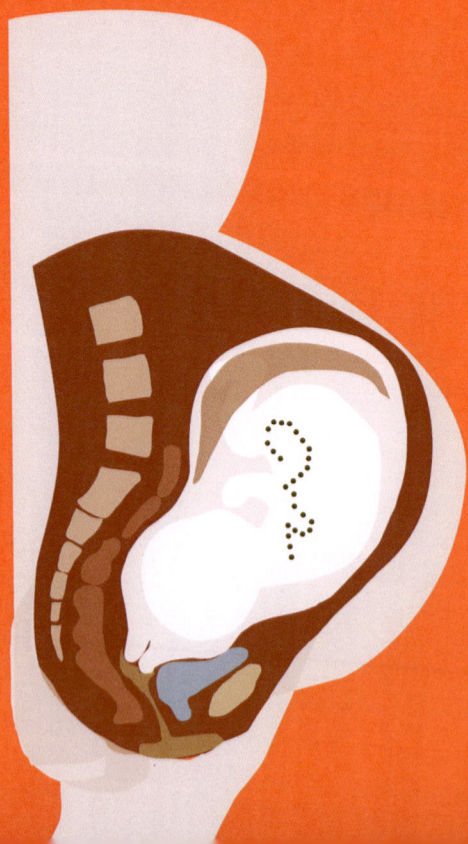

PREGNANCY MASSAGE

When you're carrying a baby or multiple babies, you have a lot of extra weight going on. Of course you do! Due to the new front load, you're likely to feel fatigued far more often. You may even notice you start to subconsciously change the way you walk, in efforts to distribute the additional body weight evenly ... hello to the prego waddle!. The way you sleep will also vary as you wriggle, roll & toss in search of a good nights sleep. On top of all of this, from day-to-day you'll need to accommodate a heavier frame... and it can be Ex-Haust-Ing.

I urge you all to do what I didn't during my first pregnancy (but did during my second) and book yourself a pregnancy massage! Whether you are 15 weeks, 20 weeks, 30 or 39! The idea of the massage is not just for a quiet lie down and a few hours of relaxation. No way. I mean it's great for those things too but the physical AND mental benefits are huge in terms of your comfort & preparation for birth.

You don't only 'deserve it' ... many of you will 'need it'. And whatever you do, don't feel guilty for taking this time for yourself. Especially if you have other littles to run around after. Pregnancy is an intense load on your body. Looking after yourself properly is sensible, safe & wise.

As a big believer in Remedial Prenatal Massage I've dedicated a whole chapter to the subject. I've called upon a brilliant remedial massage therapist, Imogen Young – owner of Remedial Massage – to take you through the importance of this particular style of massage.

When reading this chapter, I'd like to preface that nothing should be taken as advice or strict direction. Anything & everything to do with your health, your pregnancy, your baby & your birth should always be checked with your personal health practitioner.

REMEDIAL PRENATAL MASSAGE

Q. **What is Remedial Prenatal Massage?**

IY: Prenatal Remedial Massage is regular remedial massage which takes into consideration the physiological changes that occur through pregnancy, and provides a safe and appropriate treatment plan. Prenatal remedial massage utilises select soft tissue techniques to alleviate muscle tightness and pain, normalise joint ranges, reduce maternal stress and promote blood and lymphatic circulation, along with many other benefits.

Q. **How does it differ from a usual massage?**

IY: There are two key differences.

The first is the positioning of the expecting mother. After the 1st trimester, a pregnant woman cannot lie flat on her stomach or back. So, the client will usually be on her side, propped with an abundance of pillows and/or in a reclining position, again using LOTS of pillows! Front lying pregnancy pillows may be used in some circumstances. During a prenatal remedial massage there may be a few position changes but it's important for the client to know that **her comfort is essential**, and she should express any concerns she may have at any time.

The 2nd is **where** and **what** deep tissue techniques can & cannot be used. According to Traditional Chinese Medicine there are certain acupressure points that are linked to inducing labor. These acupressure points are associated with specific organs, that, when stimulated, cause an effect. For example, Large intestine 4 is located midway between the thumb and first finger, and when stimulated is suggested to promote uterine contraction and speed up the labor progress. While current research has found no clear evidence to support this, it is still advisable that deep, prolonged pressure should not be applied on these acupressure points. Other acupressure points of caution are located in the upper trap, sacrum, leg, ankle and foot. Access to certain muscles may also be challenging due to physical changes, therefore treatment of some muscles may require the client to be in a specific position or have a specific technique applied for the safe release of target tissue.

Q. What are the most common areas you treat during pregnancy?

IY: Hips and back! These two are easily the most common and it's not surprising when you think about all the changes the body is going through. In early stages of pregnancy hormones are released to relax the ligaments of the hip and lower spine, allowing for the pelvis to widen and bear a child. As the pregnancy progresses postural changes occur impacting the lower back, upper back and pelvis position. All these changes result in the muscles of the back and hips being placed under stress, and so result in discomfort.

Q. If women had to focus on one particular Trimester in terms of regular massage, which would it be and why?

IY: This is a tough one, because each pregnancy is different. Some women may experience musculoskeletal discomfort as early as the first trimester, while others may not until the late stages of pregnancy. Remedial massage CAN be performed safely throughout all stages of pregnancy. I would say that there isn't one trimester to focus on but rather when discomfort arises, it is important for pregnant women to seek help.

In saying this, physical aches and pains generally begin to occur during the second trimester. By midway through the second trimester, the impact of postural changes caused by the increasing size and weight of breasts, rib cage expansion, foetal growth and widening pelvis are beginning to be felt.

Getting on top of these aches and pains early is key to minimising discomfort throughout the pregnancy. I often recommend to my clients to receive a prenatal remedial massage at least once a month for maintenance purposes. Pregnant women should also consult with a Women's Health Physiotherapist about these aches and pains. There are many circumstances in which muscle tightness may not be the cause of pain, in which case a physio assessment is needed and massage to that area may need to be avoided. I believe it's best practice for the client if the Remedial Massage Therapist and their Physiotherapist have a close working relationship.

COMMON PREGNANCY PAINS & STRAINS

Q. In layman's terms, can you explain the reasons behind the following common pains & strains?

IY: Of course. The following list is a great place to start:

* **Hip/Pelvic Pain** – During pregnancy, hormones cause the ligaments of the pelvis to relax and stretch slightly. As a result the hip joint has a little more movement than normal, making it 'unstable'. The muscles surrounding the hip are then required to work more to help provide stability. If the muscles of the hip aren't quite strong enough, it can result in pain and tightness. Pelvic pain often presents in feelings of both sharp pains and dull aches in the back, sides and pubic region of the pelvis.

* **Lower Back Pain** – Similar to pelvic pain, lower back pain is due to hormones causing the ligaments of the spine to become slightly lax. The muscles of the lower back then have to work harder to maintain stability. In addition, the weight of the growing foetus changes your centre of gravity, your weight distribution and can change the angle of your pelvis. This in turn puts extra strain on the muscles of the back, compresses the lumbar (lower) spine and places the body in an unfamiliar posture

* **Sciatica Pain** – The sciatic is a large nerve that branches off the lumbar spine, travels through the glutes and down the legs. Sciatic pain occurs when the sciatic nerve is agitated, compressed or impinged. During pregnancy symptoms of sciatic-like pain are often caused by the postural changes associated with pregnancy and can be the result of muscular tension, sacroiliac joint (SIJ) issues, instability through the hip joint and tightness or weakness through the supporting muscle groups.

Q. How can pregnant women conquer these pains overnight when they sleep? i.e. pillow positions etc?

IY: To minimise the strain on the hip muscles when sleeping on your side, position pillows between your legs to ensure the top knee, ankle and hip are parallel. To do this, it may require using two or more pillows stacked to get the ideal height – play around with the number of pillows, their thickness and firmness. Alternatively find a side-lying pregnancy pillow that is equivalent thickness to achieve this position. Having your leg in this alignment places your hip in a neutral position, which decreases strain through the hip. If the hip is not in a neutral position, the muscles and structures at the back of the pelvis and pubic region are stretched. When you consider how many hours you sleep for at night, it's not surprising they become sore!

Understandably, this position can be challenging through the night if you like to change from side to side. If this is you, make sure you set up the same position on the other side.

LOW IMPACT EXERCISE

Q. **For low impact exercise, what do you recommend is a safe & valuable way to move the body & why?**

IY: Safe and valuable exercise is dependent on the exercise history of the individual. Recent research suggests pregnant women should try to maintain an exercise routine similar to pre-pregnancy for as long as possible. Exercise during pregnancy is important, not only for general health reasons, but also for maintaining muscle strength, stability and mobility. The goal for exercise is to maintain fitness, move without pain and provide the framework for a speedy post-pregnancy recovery.

Pilates and resistance training are great low impact options for pregnant women to move their body's and keep strong. Maintaining strength, particularly for hip and back muscles is beneficial in minimising muscular aches throughout pregnancy, as they are able to cope with the demands being placed on them. Exercise selection and intensity will need to be modified according to the individual's capabilities during the progression of pregnancy. Swimming, cycling (on exercise bike) and water walking are good options for pregnant women to maintain cardiovascular health. Exercise in the water is great for de-loading the body and reducing pain.

For women who do not have much exercise history, these options are a good place to start, but start with small durations and build gradually. It is important for all pregnant women to consult with a Women's Health Physiotherapist and/or Exercise Physiologist for their exercise routines.

Q. What exercise would you least recommend?

IY: Exercise to avoid is anything that involves a risk of falling, this can include gym exercises targeting balance, cycling or surfing. Classes that are conducted in a hot room such as 'hot yoga' and 'hot pilates' should also be avoided. Exercising in a hot environment when pregnant can increase body temperature too much and risk fainting or light-headedness.

High impact exercises should be monitored according to the individual's pregnancy and exercise history. Typically early into the second semester high impact exercises, such as running, will become uncomfortable and at this point it is recommended to stop. High impact exercises can place excessive stress and strain on the pelvic floor and hip stabilising muscles potentially leading to inflammation, pain and injury to muscles, ligaments and other soft tissue.

Women should consult with their Women's Health Physiotherapist and/or Exercise Physiologist about their exercise routines, as they vary from individual to individual.

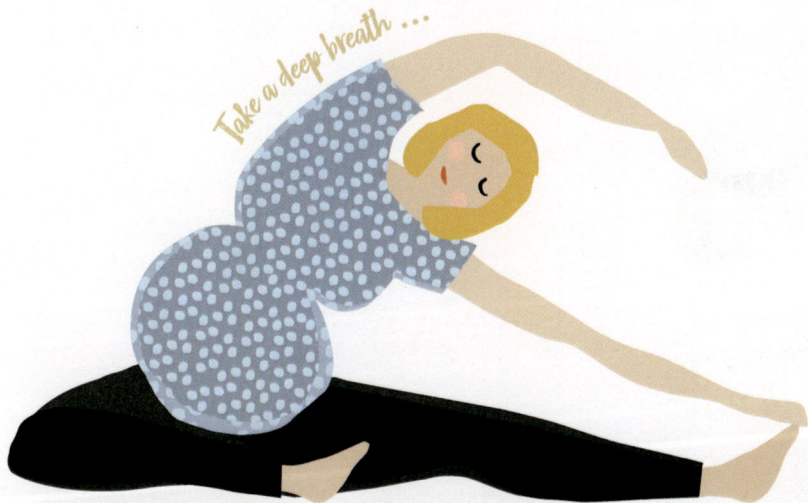

Q. Is there a daily stretch pregnant women can practise to relieve some of the main areas we feel pain i.e. hips, lower back and pelvis?

IY: Of course! Personally I would move through these stretches to make more of a flow, ~40-60 seconds per stretch 2-3x through.

1. **With chair:**
   * Seated glute stretch
   * Hamstring forward bend with chair

2. **Floor stretches:**
   * Pigeon pose
   * Hip flexor stretch (kneeling lunge)
   * Thread the needle
   * Cat-cows
   * Child's pose

Q. If there was 1 or a few items i.e. a foam roller, a bolster, tennis ball, resistance band, fit ball etc to invest in during pregnancy, what would your top tip be?

IY: I would recommend a foam roller for a bit of self release work and a resistance band for strengthening exercises! I would also recommend investing in looking after yourself and your body during pregnancy. This can be through finding a form of exercise that you enjoy and can do throughout the pregnancy, getting regular massage and giving yourself timeout.

REMEDIAL MASSAGE AND INDUCTION

Q. For women entering their 40th or 41st week ... can Remedial Massage help to naturally induce labor ?

IY: This is an interesting topic, as there are mixed views around it. As I mentioned earlier, there are acupressure points located in the body that are believed to be linked to inducing labor. This form of treatment has been around for centuries and many women and therapists swear by it. However there is little clinical evidence to support its efficacy. If women would like to try this method I would strongly suggest they speak with their medical team and to seek out a therapist who is trained and experienced in acupressure, particularly for labor induction. Remedial massage or relaxation massage however CAN be beneficial in relaxing the mother by promoting activation of the parasympathetic nervous system.

HIGH RISK PREGNANCIES AND REMEDIAL MASSAGE

Q. Is there ever a circumstance where Remedial Massage should be avoided? i.e. for mums on best rest, is massage out of the question? If so, why?

IY: For high risk pregnancies it is advisable to consult your medical team before using any additional or alternative therapies. Generally, Prenatal Remedial Massage should be avoided for high risk pregnancies, unless advised otherwise by a medical professional. There are a number of pregnancy complications that are considered high-risk and can result in a mother being placed on bed rest. Massage is not advised when there is a risk to the mother or baby's life.

In cases where the obstetrician or midwife has advised that prenatal massage would be suitable, then a light 30 minute massage can be performed in a side-lying position.

Q. For pregnant women also carrying toddlers or small children, should they be applying the same "lifting techniques" we are always taught i.e. bend from the knees?

IY: Yes, use your legs and glutes to lift (NOT your back) – lower to a squat position and keep your back as neutral as possible. Also, try not to favour one side when carrying young children, it is good to try and keep the body as even as possible. By favouring one side it can lead to tightness and additional discomfort.

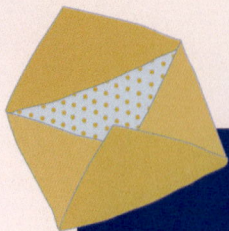

A Letter to Her Pregnant Self

FROM KLAIRE

This mother, Klaire carried twins! Two wonderful little people who now reflect their darling mother & her warm, bright nature. To grow two in one body is an almighty power. A beautiful gift. A wild & wonderful journey. Klaires future includes a harmony of cooes and giggles … incredible. Simply incredible.

Klaire writes back in time to offer herself words of comfort, wisdom & joy.

Dear me,

First up, you are doing amazing sweetie.

You are growing two humans. Growing all their little fingers and toes, their little organs and eyelashes. You are doing that. So give yourself a break. No literally! Have a break. Put down the laptop, leave the laundry, don't worry about dinner. Lay down, have a bath, have a cup of tea. Not only do you NEED it right now but also you won't get any of that very soon. So while you are freaking out trying to get everything ready for your babies (and lets be real, a large portion of what you are freaking out about is irrreeeeleevantttt), realise your babies are already here and you are already giving them everything. So it's ok to slow down and just be the incubator you currently are.

Honestly, most of the things you are freaking out about needing, you won't need before they are born and if you forget anything someone will be more then happy to head to a store to pick it up for you if it means they get to meet the bundles of joy.

Take that break, slow down. Not long from now those two little rascals will make their entrance much earlier than expected (but a bit early it always somewhat expected in multiples), and you'll spend two months at the hospital. So if you wont rest for you, do it for those babies. Less stress & more relaxing will give them the best chance of staying put that bit longer.

But if they do make a dramatic entrance before their cue, don't worry. You will be scared, you will be worried about them. But it will all be ok. They will start off weighing just a tiny 1.5kg each. They'll be size of your palm with tubes everywhere and monitors beeping around them ... but not long after they will be boisterous bundles of energy, kicking and punching as hard as they do inside you.

Enjoy that feeling of EIGHT limbs poking into every corner of your organs. Enjoy the TWENTY fingers grabbing and prodding your insides. Enjoy that feeling when they wriggle and move and you can't work out if it was Twin A or Twin B!

Someone once told you that how they behave in utero is likely to reflect their personalities. You'll spend the whole pregnancy thinking your little girl is the wriggler ... but oh you were wrong! Turns out it's your little boys legs ... kick, kick kicking!

One of the hardest things of pregnancy is that it's only you. You can't ask your partner or your mum's opinion. If something feels off or the movements don't seem right, no one else can tell you (except those with fancy machines), so don't feel bad going to the doctor or the hospital when you feel it to be necessary. The medical staff are always so accommodating, and your peace of mind and knowing that everything is ok, is all that matters. There are two babies within your body and you have every right to do what you need to do, to know they are safe. You will spend the rest of your life advocating for them. That job starts now.

Remember that first scan? Two babies! I mean who would have thought!?! Especially as there aren't twins anywhere in the family. Turns out it's not always genetic! It will take you weeks to wrap your head around it. Lying awake at night thinking about all the important questions like, 'Do they take two presents or one to a birthday party?" And, 'What if you can't tell them apart?" But none of that will matter. They will be their own little people and you just figure it all out as it happens.

Your biggest fear is this, What if you don't have enough love for both of them? How can you give your whole self when there are two? If motherhood is hard with one, surely you won't be able to be a good mum when there are two babies screaming for your attention?

All the things you are worried about will never cross your mind again.

When these monkeys come out, they will have already had months of being cuddled up together, beating each other up ... their innate bond has been there right from the start. But I know you are worried about your bond with them. Will you feel it straight away?

All those Hollywood scenes flash in your mind, where the love is bursting out between the mum and her newborn. You know what? You might not get that ... and that's ok!! In fact, you most likely won't get that feeling as soon as you meet them. You'll be handed these tiny, gooey little people. You've never met them. You are high on endorphins and medication. It's ok in this moment to not feel much at all.

Remember, you're the person that took years to say, 'I love you' to your partner. So perhaps it seems unlikely to feel the rush of love to begin ...but again, that is ok. It could take time. But don't feel embarrassed or fear that the bond will never come, because you have a whole lifetime! ... But guess what? Your heart will expand every single day as it fills up with their smiles & their laughter.

But enough worrying about when they are earthside... especially between the nausea, the discomfort and the 'trying' to enjoy the pregnancy. For now, take a million photos! Photos of that belly & of the amazing things your body is doing. You might feel gross, you might feel huge! But take the photos ok? You don't have to show anyone or do anything with them... but to have them there so that one day you can look back and remember, it's your Jess and Leo in there.

So snap away. Take a photo every week & right from the early days because you never know when those little pumpkins will decide it's time to come out.

... and then all of a sudden as if like magic, you aren't pregnant anymore. And who knows ... you may never have that big, swollen belly again.

On another note... everyone will have advice for you. EVERYONE! The old man in the line at the supermarket, everyone who's had a kid or been near a kid in their lifetime, your mum's sisters friend. It's funny how society thinks they own a pregnant body isn't it? And the amount of times people ask you if it was IVF when they find out its twins! In what world is that OK!?

But of course, there's some advice offered that did actually help. So here it is, for you:

1. Only take advice from parents with multiples. It's just a whole different beast. Parents in the same boat are the most efficient people in the world. Triplet mum advice?! It is pure gold!

2. Make sure to visit a Women's Health Physio. Find one you like and just book it in! All the information you hear about the pelvic floor and Kegel exercises etc ... turns out to be the exact opposite of what's needed in your personal case. Go figure! You are currently overacting your pelvic floor needs, so for the benefit of your post pregnancy body and her recovery ... a Women's Health Physio is a necessity.

3. Don't take anyone's advice (I get the irony).

On that note, pour yourself another cup of tea, get in a warm bath and enjoy those squirming inside feelings as twin A and Twin B somersault.

... because soon enough they won't be Twin A and Twin B, they will be your Jess and Leo. And then the real adventure begins.

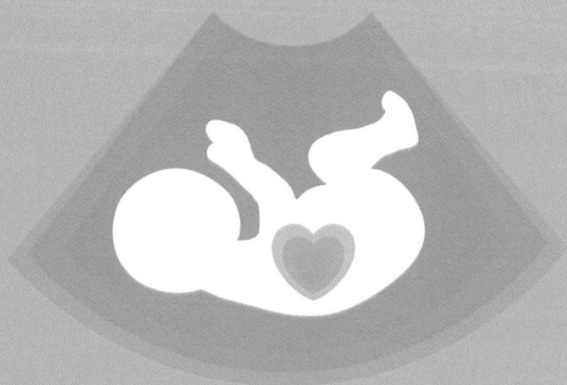

PREGNANCY SCANS

Scans during pregnancy... some of us love them! Others find them terrifying. Regardless of your feelings however, there are a particular set of scans in Australia that will occur over the 9months. Confused about what they are all for? I don't doubt! That's why I've welcomed Danielle Paterson, a talented Diagnostic Medical Sonographer based in WA (who by the way, did one of my scans during my second pregnancy!), to walk us through the subject.

It should be noted that some women will require more scans than are mentioned below. This may be for an array of reasons (I had so many more during my first pregnancy as Hamish was aways measuring on the smaller side), but for the most part the explanations below should apply.

DATING SCAN

Usually the Dating Scan occurs at the 8 week mark, as this is a perfect time for this scan.

8 weeks is of course not always achievable - and sometimes it needs to be brought forward. Reasons for this can include a complex previous pregnancy history/ unreliable last menstrual period dates/spotting/pain/bleeding during early pregnancy). For these reasons it's always best to trust your GP regarding at what point you should have your Dating Scan.

Remember your pregnancy is totally unique.It is not a case of 'one size fits all.'

The aim of the dating scan is not only to "date" the pregnancy but to ensure the pregnancy is intra-uterine, a heart beat is present and to determine how many babies are present. During this scan, the uterus and the ovaries are also assessed to take note of any potential issues for a progressing pregnancy.

12 WEEK SCAN

This scan is usually not compulsory. You may opt for it for personal reasons or it may be recommended by your GP, particularly if you are in the high risk or geriatric category.

If the reason for the "12 week ultrasound" is for prenatal aneuploidy screening (i.e. to check for chromosomal abnormality), there are now 2 main, non invasive methods of screening;

Method 1: The Nuchal translucency ultrasound is part of the first trimester screen. This looks at the normal fluid-filled subcutaneous space behind the neck of the foetus during the late 1st trimester and early 2nd trimester (11 weeks 3 days to 13 weeks 6 days).

Method 2: If you are having the non-invasive prenatal testing (NIPT) then you will need an "early anatomy scan." NIPT is currently the most reliable screening test available for detecting chromosomal abnormalities Trisomy 21, 13 and 18, determining gender and a range of other potential abnormalities. The "early anatomy scan" is ideally done between 13 and 14 weeks when the baby is a little bigger. The "early anatomy ultrasound" does not alleviate the need for an "anatomy / morphology ultrasound."

ANATOMY/ANOMALY/MORPHOLOGY SCAN

This is the "20 week ultrasound."

This ultrasound is ideally done between 19 and 21 weeks. Here, we look in detail at the anatomical make-up of the foetus, the placenta, umbilical cord, amniotic fluid and, last but not least, the uterus, cervix and ovaries of the mother. This is typically the longest scan! The level of time required is often determined by the level of cooperation from baby!

Q. Why might other scans be required during pregnancy?

DP: Depending on your antenatal care team and a multitude of factors in pregnancy, many women will have at least 1 third trimester ultrasound. Some women will have cervical length ultrasounds and others will need extra scans if they have a complex pregnancy or health history.

Q. For multiples (twins, triplets etc), is the scanning process more difficult?

DP: The rules for ultrasound in multiple pregnancy are very different to that of a single pregnancy. The type of twins or triplets determines the frequency of scans. Even in the most straightforward multiple pregnancy, there are many extra ultrasounds.

Naturally, multiple pregnancy is automatically associated with more types of complications than a single pregnancy and therefore more needs to be monitored to ensure everything is going smoothly. As you would expect, the more babies the longer each scan takes!

Q. What is the difference between an Abdominal Scan & a Vaginal Scan?

DP: **Transabdominal ultrasound** (Abdominal Scan) is performed on top of the skin, using the semi-full bladder as a "window" to see the uterus and baby.

Transvaginal ultrasound (Vaginal Scan) is performed by placing an ultrasound probe just inside the vagina, in order to have a closer, more detailed look at the gynaecological organs and the pregnancy.

Q. Why do some women require both?

DP: Sometimes after starting with a transabdominal ultrasound it becomes apparent the imaging is not adequate through the abdomen.

Consequently a closer view is needed and a transvaginal approach will be required. It really does sound worse than it is, and the greater detail obtained with this type of scan makes it all worthwhile.

Q. Can ultrasounds pick up physical abnormalities with baby?

DP: The idea behind antenatal ultrasound is to ensure everything is as it should be, so ideally, yes physical abnormalities will be detected. Examination quality is affected by multiple factors including but not limited to, gestational age and maternal body habitus. In a perfect world all physical abnormalities would be detected but sometimes they are extremely small or subtle or do not manifest until a later stage in pregnancy.

Q. It's recommended that women drink water prior to their scan & hold in a wee. For those who suffer shocking sickness during pregnancy and are unable to keep any fluids down on the day of their appointment, can a scan still be performed?

DP: We can always see from a woman's 'green-ness' as they walk through the doors that drinking & holding water is going to be a struggle. We of course, understand completely. If you can be hydrated and hang on, great. If you can't, it may just mean a transvaginal ultrasound approach will be necessary.

Q. Are there particular questions women should ask during their scans i.e. is it important that mum knows what she's looking at? Working out what's what can be very confusing!

DP: First time mums and dads rarely see what we are talking about, even after pointing it out to them. That's normal. There's a reason it takes such a long time to train as a sonographer, most of us saw the moon initially too!

Hopefully you get a sonographer who patiently points things out and explains as they scan. If they don't, you can absolutely ask them to show you 'the cute things' when possible. Bear in mind however that the foetal heart, brain and spine can often be complex to assess & your sonographer may likely need to focus harder, perhaps silently, as they scan these parts.

Q. If during a scan, there is an unfortunate situation where no heartbeat is detected, what are the next steps?

DP: These situations never get easier or less upsetting ... even for a sonographer who is scanning someone they've never met.

The absence of a heartbeat means the pregnancy has ended.

9 times out of 10 you will be told there is no heartbeat (many parents will actually notice themselves during the screen). Typically at this point, your referring doctor will be notified immediately and a care plan will be formulated. The gestational age at the time of pregnancy failure will determine the management path.

Q. For women who are pregnant and who are yet to have their first scan, it can be quite an anxious wait - especially for those who have lost babies in the past. From your experience as a sonographer do you have any words of wisdom to ease this angst?

* Firstly, remember you are not alone. Unfortunately so many women go through the hell of pregnancy failure and infertility. Lean on those around you for support as talking is so important. A lot of the time you will be so surprised by who can empathise. This may help you breathe a little easier.

* Choose a GP/OB/Antenatal team that you assess to be caring and empathetic. A team you are confident and comfortable will manage your mental health as well as your pregnancy as best as possible.

* Blood tests will be done quite soon after determining you are pregnant and then after the dating scan. Whilst 8 weeks is ideal for a dating scan, you can always come slightly earlier if your doctor deems it a good idea to help with anxiety levels. If you have a history of pregnancy loss, discuss with your doctor the possibility of more frequent ultrasounds.

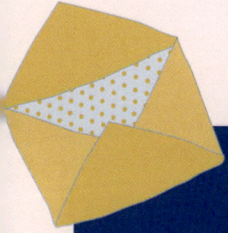

A Letter to Her Pregnant Self

FROM CLAIRE

This mother, Clare, climbed mountains to meet her baby. An IVF journey that tested a woman in a way she shouldn't have to be tested. How you may ask? Well …

2 and a 1/2 long years, 7 egg collection surgeries + anaesthetics, 10 IVF rounds/transfers, 100+ blood tests, 60+ ultrasounds, 500+ needles, 100+ bruises, supplements, medications and plenty of side effects. 803 days of trying to conceive, 1 early miscarriage,1 ED visit and scare …

A test? Yes. But my oh my … did she pass with flying colours. A rainbow now sleeps in her arms & giggles during her every day. She met her child. She is now mother.

Clare (@claire_ridley) writes to her pregnant self in a way that is honest & courageous. She fills her future with joyful anticipation that will hopefully resonate with anyone reading, who is walking a similar road on the way to meet their baby. May that day come, may it come soon & may it bring such loveliness.

Dear me,

'If I knew what I know now'

If I knew what I know now, I'd know it was always going to be my baby boy.

I'd know that he'd be perfect and my greatest ever creation.

I'd know that I was missing a piece of my heart for 39 years.

I'd know that my life was never going to be the same ever again and my heart would be finally completely full the day he arrived.

I'd know why it was worth every second of the three years I waited for him arrive.

I'd know every blood test, needle, ultrasound and procedure were a walk in the park compared to the thought of never meeting him.

I'd know to stay calm and relax and be at peace with the IVF process and journey because it would make me the stronger, more patient and resilient person I am today.

I'd know there was no need to stress about being a good mother and to listen to my heart and not get overwhelmed by the mountains of advice given as soon as you fall pregnant.

I'd also know that a lot of that advice would also come in so handy and that I'd absorb more of it than I'd realise.

I'd know that the advice and information would also be very important in advocating for my IVF treatments, my health and my baby's health.

I'd know that he'd be the perfect addition to our family and bring us all closer together than ever before.

I'd know that my relationship would be stronger and create a very special new bond between my husband and I that would connect us all.

I'd know that birth was nothing to stress about all my life and in fact it would be one of the most empowering, positive, surprisingly calm and enjoyable life experiences I have ever had.

I'd know that the sleepless nights, the aches, the pains didn't last long and I'd go through all of that again to experience the precious newborn stage again.

I'd know that waking up in the middle of the night to that tiny bundle of joy would make anything I feared about the lack of sleep seem insignificant.

I'd know that my career is still important but it is not important enough to miss out on experiencing motherhood and that there is room for both in my life.

I'd know to take more photos and videos because even though my camera roll has 20,000 photos, I'd take more because time flies faster than any one told you it would.

I'd know that I would chill out more about life being so perfect because in an instant you can't control all the things you used to and those things that used to be important just aren't anymore.

I'd know that I can still be a fun mum and still enjoy the things I used to like going out for dinners and travelling and that I wouldn't have to give those things up completely.

I'd know that doing the things I used to enjoy are now even more fulfilling as I get to experience them with my baby boy.

I'd know it would finally my turn to take him to see Santa, to get to 'be' Santa and the Easter Bunny and to really experience the magic of these holidays that children bring.

I'd know it would finally be my turn to host birthday parties, to post my 'first smile, first day of school' pics and not feel sad when everyone else did.

I'd know some days would be tough, there would be tears, days in bed and exhaustion but none of that would compare to the tears, the pain, the exhaustion and that longing for a child and IVF and infertility brings.

I'd know that IVF would rob me of so much – the surprise of falling pregnant, old-fashioned baby making, time, money and my mental health but I would know that IVF would also give me the greatest blessing and all of it was infinitely worth it.

I'd know that positivity, perseverance and tenacity were three of the most important traits I have and without them I may not have ended up with my baby in my arms today.

I'd know that during everything I endured there was always hope and throughout life I will always have hope.

If I knew what I know now, I would know that being a mother and having a child is truly the greatest gift you can ever receive and one that I will never ever take for granted.

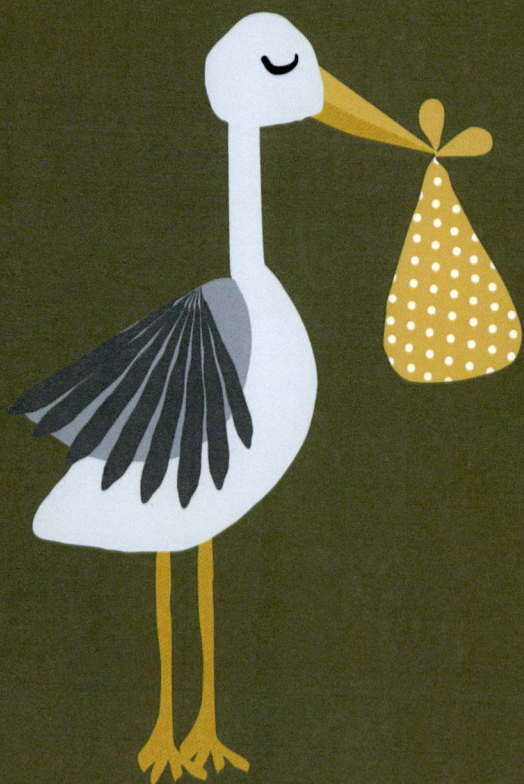

THE
NEWBORN
CRY

Why is this a chapter? May seem a little odd perhaps? Well funnily enough, this is the chapter I felt as though the book HAD TO HAVE. It was not going to print without. It's my way of 'paying it forward' to all mums in the hope it will help prepare you & keep you on the calmer side of frazzled moments with bub.

This subject *needs* its own chapter because the sound of your baby crying is what might un-do you. Why? You'll find out soon enough.

You can prepare for a lot of the motherhood journey while you're pregnant. Within reason. You can read all the books (thanks for choosing mine PS!), you can listen to all the podcasts (my fav is Beyond The Bump PPS), you can attend all the classes & you can watch a million episodes of One Born Every Minute (I was an ADDICT during my first pregnancy PPPS)... but whatever you read, watch or listen to is not going to be your reality.

Upon reflection, what you can't plan for is how the sound of your baby's cry will affect you. Your baby's unique cry will have a particular frequency that only you, their mother, will hear. And holy moly, it may challenge you.

This chapter isn't meant to frighten anyone as, after all, crying is just bubs way of communicating. And trust me – babies are smart and very in-tune with their emotions from the moment they're born. Crying can mean many things (hunger, wind, tiredness, general discomfort, boredom, pain – or it can simply be their way of saying 'Oi mum, pick me up!') Crying can be helpful as it helps us meet their needs, without too much guesswork.

It's the sound of the occasional ballistic cry that might send you over the edge. And I'm not talking about a colic-y bub. It's not a sob or a squeal. It's not a yelp or a whisper. It's the hysterical, uncontrollable cry that gets you. For me personally, the sound of my baby crying like this is the most challenging part of parenting to date.

This chapter is designed to help you prepare for something that you MAY find as tough as I do. Remember though, you may not! And if not, oh my good gracious, I am green with envy!

To help cope with this 'hysteria' for like of-a-better-term, I needed to look beyond western medicine & physical activity. Beyond the apps & other forms of cutting edge technology such as The Snow. I needed to bring in the BIG GUN ... Mindfulness.

You need to understand & get comfortable with this word before laboring & parenting a newborn baby. 'Mindfulness' is not a wishy-washy/new age term. It is a little magic trick, that, when used wisely, timely & correctly, can give you the ability to cope.

Here we welcome Stephanie Johnson to take over. Stephanie is a qualified Health and Wellness Specialist with a heap of experience in this space.

Fun fact, Steph is also my sister-in-law, and aunty to my boys! Throughout both of my pregnancies she's given me the gift of yoga, breath & stillness. I am of course a huge advocate for her knowledge & expert talents, and I'm very fortunate to now share them with you all.

Before I pass over the mic, if this aspect of parenting concerns you (i.e. crying & loud noises in general,) then to try and prepare yourself you could practice the exercises Steph is about to walk us through, while playing something you find uncomfortable to listen to, or to be in the presence of. For example a super loud TV or irritating music i.e. Cocomelon or death metal. Both equally rage inducing.

Please Refrain from putting these exercises into motion if you are already finding your pregnancy exhausting or stressful, as you don't want to add any extra pressure on yourself. And most importantly check any new exercises with your medical team first, especially if you have a medical condition and have been advised to rest & keep your heart rate steady.

If you are hungry to challenge your mental strength in times of extreme discomfort – go mumma! I wish I had taught myself earlier on.

Steph, take it away! Save Our Sanity!

Steph (SJ) ... 'There is nothing more essential to our health and wellbeing than breathing; take air in, let it out, repeat. Yet, as a species, humans have lost the ability to breathe correctly. By making the slightest adjustment to the way we inhale and exhale, we can restore our physical and mental health, balance our nervous system, and improve, shift and change our mood. An adult at rest breathes about 17,280 to 23,040 times a day at 12 to 16 breaths per minute.'

Q. What is deep breathing? How can it affect our mood?

SJ: There are two phases of breathing: inhaling (taking a breath in) and exhalation (breathing out). When you inhale, the diaphragm contracts and moves downwards. This creates space in the chest cavity and the lungs expand into it. When you exhale, the diaphragm relaxes as the amount of air in the lungs is reduced.

In most cases we're not breathing properly. If our breath is shallow, we can be imposing stress on the body or the stress we feel may be contributing to shallow breathing. Deep breathing naturally slows the breath down. It requires you to relax your abdomen while you take a deep breath in. By breathing deeply we are slowly filling the lungs with air and allowing the lungs to expand, which will move the diaphragm. At the exhale we release all the air out as the diaphragm relaxes and the chest wall recoils. In focusing our awareness on this process, we slow our breathing pattern which can create a physiological change in our body altering our mood and how we feel.

Q. Is deep breathing a form of meditation? If not, how do they differ?

SJ: Deep breathing is an entry point to becoming more mindful and practicing acceptance. Our breath is the one true thing that is present in the moment. By paying attention to our breath, we develop the strength and awareness of mindfulness. Through mindfulness and becoming aware of our breath, we start to notice the space in between our breath and our thoughts which can lead us into deep states of meditation.

DEEP BREATHING 101

Phase 1

1. Sit in a chair or cross-legged and upright on the floor and relax the shoulders
2. Place one hand over the navel and slowly breathe into the belly. You should feel the belly expand with each breath in, deflate with each breath out. Practice this a few times.
3. Next, move the hand up a few inches so that it's covering the bottom of the rib cage. Focus the breath into the location of the hand, expanding the ribs with each inhale, retracting them with each exhale. Practice this for about three to five breaths.
4. Move the hand to just below the collarbone. Breathe deeply into this area and imagine the chest spreading out and withdrawing with each exhale. Do this for a few breaths.

Phase 2

1. Connect all these motions into one breath, inhale into the stomach, lower rib cage, then chest.
2. Exhale in the opposite direction, first emptying the chest, then the rib cage, then the stomach. Feel free to use a hand and feel each area as you breathe in and out of it
3. Continue this same sequence for about a dozen rounds. These motions may feel very awkward at first, but after a few breaths will get easier.

Q. When there is noise that heightens a feeling of panic, frustration or discomfort – what can we do to help us sit within these moments & hold a sense of calm & composure?

SJ: The mind & body are often disconnected. The breath in all its subtleness bridges the metaphysical relationship between mind and matter, between substance and attribute, and between potentiality and actuality. Everything affects the breath and everything starts and ends with the breath.

As Viktor Frankl, author of "Man's Search for Meaning" so beautifully articulates, in between the stimulus and response there is a space and in that space is our power to choose our response. The stimulus here is the noise and our response is the feeling of panic, frustration and discomfort. As a result of this response we experience a physiological effect in our body. Our heart rate starts to increase, our breathing pattern quickens and in turn our feelings of panic and frustration subside.

By practicing deep breathing regularly it increases our awareness of our response. In moments of panic and frustration, it's important to come back to your breath, recognise how you're responding and consciously choose how you wish to respond. This is empowering.

Q. Or, can we learn to silence this surrounding noise, i.e. and unsettled baby?

SJ: The more we practice the above techniques, the more we will become experienced at learning to quieten (not silence) the surrounding noise. There's a beautiful fable about two wolves, also known as "The Wolves Within". It's a story about a grandfather explaining his inner conflicts and struggles to his grandson.

An old Cherokee told his grandson, "My son, there is a battle between two wolves inside us all. One is Evil. It is anger, jealousy, greed, resentment, inferiority, lies and ego, The other is Good. It is joy, peace, love, hope, humility, kindness, empathy and truth" The boy thought about it, and asked "Grandfather, which wolf wins?" The old man quietly replied "The one you feed".

The story highlights the capacity we all have as individuals to place our attention on what we choose to strengthen. We can choose our response in any given situation. We can't silence a noise but the more we practice certain things, the easier it will be to turn our attention to these things.

Q. **When a room becomes swollen with an uncomfortable silence – are there techniques that can enable us to sit calmly in silence, rather than filling the space with unwanted tension or passive conversation? For example when there is an awkward or tense 'vibe' between new parents OR a mum with her newborn + other children.**

SJ: The following exercise is known as Box Breathing. Navy SEALS use this technique to stay calm and focused in tense situations. It's simple.

BOX BREATHING EXERCISE

1. Inhale to a count of 4; hold 4; exhale 4; hold 4. Repeat. Longer exhalations will elicit a stronger parasympathetic response. A variation of box breathing to more deeply relax the body that's especially effective before sleeping is as follows:
2. Inhale to a count of 4; hold 4; exhale 6; hold 2. Repeat – try at last six rounds, more if necessary.

Q. **Postpartum rage can be intensely overwhelming and lead to crippling guilt and shame. There will be moments when a new mum may feel as though she's on the cusp of snapping. Is there a breathing technique (or any other technique), that can help to redirect this 'rage'?**

The following breathing technique has been scientifically proven to lower heart rate, blood pressure and sympathetic stress. It helps the mind to become still and tranquil, which further eradicates problems like stress and anxiety.This effective breathing technique is great to use when you feel yourself getting stressed, before going to sleep or when trying to settle a crying baby.

TECHNIQUE 1

1. Hand Positioning: Place the thumb of your right hand gently over your right nostril and the ring finger of the same hand on the left nostril. The forefinger and middle finger should rest between the eyebrows.
2. Close the right nostril with the thumb and inhale through the left nostril very slowly
3. At the top of the breath, pause briefly, holding both nostrils closed, then lift just the thumb to exhale through the right nostril.
4. At the natural conclusion of the exhale, hold both nostrils closed for a moment, then inhale through the right nostril.
5. Continue alternating breaths through the nostrils for five to ten cycles.

Q. Sleeping ... and hearing those haunting 'phantom cries' i.e. when you 'think' you hear the baby stir/cry. Is there a way we can allow our minds to release this sense of anticipation & relax into a deeper sleep?

The following technique made famous by Dr. Andrew Weil places the body into a state of deep relaxation which will allow the mind to release the sense of anticipation and relax into a deeper sleep.

TECHNIQUE 2

1. Take a breathe in, then exhale through your mouth with a whoosh sound.
2. Close the mouth and inhale quietly through your noise to a mental count of four.
3. Hold for a count of seven.
4. Exhale completely through your mouth, with a whoosh, to the count of eight.
5. Repeat this cycle for at least four breaths.

Dr Weil offers a step-by-step instructional on YouTube, which has been viewed more than five million times. Have a look, it's very worth it!

1. Start to become aware of your physical body.
2. Notice areas in your body that are becoming increasingly tight and stressed. This might be in your belly, your shoulders, your jaw, your mouth.
3. Consciously start to relax these parts of your body (What you're strengthening is the ability to create space between the crippling sound and your actual response).

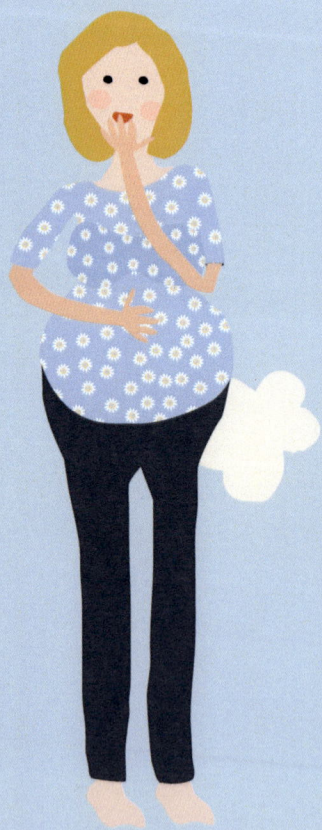

TABOO • TABOO • TABOO • TABOO • TABOO

TABOO

TABOO • TABOO • TABOO • TABOO • TABOO

The notion of 'taboo' is probably my favourite element to explore on the subject of pregnancy & birth. There are so many nitty-gritty elements to cover! Unfortunately many of them (too many of them) have the ability to make us feel unnecessarily awkward, embarrassed, shy and/or just a little icky. Right?

Well … there is NO NEED! Your body, however it may behave as you grow human life, is an incredibly intuitive, wise and able vessel. It is strong, as are you.

Having said this, of course, there are always going to be queries and wonders that dance around in your thoughts. Let's be real. Every pregnant woman is going to type something into her Google search, while hiding under the sheets late at night. We're all human, and we're all curious folk. And to be fair, we all exercise various levels of dignity, right?

So don't get too overwhelmed by Dr Google and all of his insidious links. Hopefully the list of "private" queries below, along with the explanations, will resolve some of your curiosities. Erin Phibbs – Midwife, Birth Educator and the founder of The Birth Trust (@thebirthtrust) – has very kindly embraced the theme of this chapter by providing oodles of information & insight.

I cannot recommend following The Birth Trust more highly if you're pregnant or if you're a mum! I am obsessed with Erin's content! It's realistic, informative, relatable, reliable and it articulately leans into her wealth of knowledge & experience in the pregnancy, birth & postpartum space.

Erin, Please Explain;

LET'S CHAT

Q. Increased Vaginal Discharge

EP: Hormones play a huge role in the bodily changes we experience during pregnancy. A higher level of Estrogen during pregnancy, especially during the first and third trimester, commonly results in an increase in vaginal discharge.

As if intense fatigue, all day sickness and sore boobs isn't enough, there are also soggy knickers to deal with!

Milky white discharge is normal. This white-ish clear and mild smelling discharge is medically known as Leukorrhea. Higher levels of Estrogen increase the blood flow to the pelvic organs and cause the mucous membranes to work in overdrive, leading to the production of more discharge than you might otherwise be used to.

The hormones don't just stop there. While Estrogen may thin and cause a discharge surplus, progesterone thickens it. It's not uncommon for women to notice discharge becoming thicker and stickier during the late stages of pregnancy.

Q. Frequent Farting. Why do women produce so much more gas than usual?

EP: At the risk of sounding like a broken record, this common pregnancy symptom is also the result of hormones. Higher levels of Progesterone support your pregnancy, which is great, right? However, Progesterone relaxes the muscles throughout your body, including your intestinal muscles. This leads to a slowing down of digestion and a build up of gas. Bloating, burping and frequent farting are common complaints of pregnant women, and their partners too.

Q. Vulvar Varicosities ... the cause/need to worry/any prevention?

EP: Varicosities or varicose veins as they're more commonly known, occur when a vein becomes enlarged, dilated, twisted or overfilled with blood. Vulva varicosities are varicose veins that develop on the vulva. It's estimated that between 4 and 10 percent of pregnant women will develop vulva varicosities.

The three major physiological changes that occur during pregnancy that increase the chances of developing varicose veins are; increased blood volume, pressure on the Inferior Vena Cava (the largest vein in your body) and pregnancy hormones that cause vein walls to become less rigid. Most women who experience vulva varicosities report similar symptoms, such as:

* Heaviness, pressure or pain in the vulva
* Pressure or pain in the vulva that gets worse after exercise, prolonged standing and sexual activity
* Swelling and/or itching of the vulva

To avoid exacerbating symptoms try wearing support garments, engaging in regular light exercise, manage excessive weight gain and avoid prolonged periods of standing or walking. Applying ice to the affected area and resting horizontally are great ways to manage the uncomfortable symptoms of vulva varicosities. The good news is that vulva varicosities typically disappear, without any treatment, after birth.

Q. Swollen Vulva?

EP: Unfortunately swelling in pregnancy isn't reserved for the feet and ankles alone. A swollen vulva is a common symptom of pregnancy and can appear as early as 1 month after conception. Blood flow, blood volume and hormones can be blamed for almost all the uncomfortable, and sometimes embarrassing, symptoms of pregnancy. In the case of your swollen vulva, this is true. Increased blood flow to the area causes swelling, as well as the pressure from your ever-growing uterus. Increased blood flow to the pelvic region during pregnancy supports the growth of your baby, but may also cause swelling and a change of colour of your vulva. You may notice that your labia are a deeper darker colour than usual.

Q. Fears around pooping/farting during birth?

EP: I've still yet to meet someone that feels ok about the idea of pooing in plain sight of others, especially in front of strangers. The fear of pooing during birth is close to the top of most women's 'please-don't-let-it-happen-to-me' list. While it's not something anyone wants to do, it is something that all maternity care providers are accustomed to. I'd say it's commonplace in birth settings around the world.

You may be embarrassed about the thought now, but I assure you that in the moment you likely won't even notice.

For some people, understanding why it occurs and reframing it as a positive, before labor begins, can really help them to fully surrender and not hold back during birth. Your birth canal and rectum are parallel to one another, as your baby's head descends, anything that's in the rectum will be pushed out too. So, focus on that, trust your midwife's sensitivity and be reassured that if and when it happens your baby is not far behind it.

Q. Outrageously high sex drive?

EP: In my experience there are two extremes when it comes to pregnancy libido. You either couldn't think of anything worse or you're hornier than hell. If you're experiencing the latter and you want to know why, keep reading.

Many changes during pregnancy can lead to a higher than usual libido. Again, we can thank our hormones for this one. Higher levels of human placental lactogen (hPL), Estrogen, Progesterone and Testosterone make some women feel extra sexy. You might find that your vulva becomes engorged and more sensitive due to increased blood flow. Some women feel embarrassed by their engorged vulva, but think of it this way, it's essentially a vulval erection. Enjoy it.

The end of the 'whenever we want it' spontaneity is looming, so if you're looking for it, here's your permission to embrace the changes and get down and dirty while you can.

It would be remiss of me not to mention that for some women, sex can lead to uterine contractions. This happens in response to increased levels of Oxytocin. Breast and nipple stimulation, orgasms and semen are all to blame. This doesn't mean that the horizontal tango should be off the agenda, it's just a reminder that if you feel any pain, discomfort or experience any signs or symptoms of labor check in with your care provider.

Q. Can a baby feel or be hurt by partner's penis during sex?

EP: There are men all over the world that believe their penis to be so large that it will touch the baby during sex … I think a brief anatomy lesson is needed to clear this one up.

During pregnancy the baby grows inside the amniotic sac, which is housed within the uterus. The neck of the uterus is called the cervix. During pregnancy the cervix is long and closed and the opening to the cervix creates a clever little thing called the mucous plug. During penetrative sex, when a penis enters the vagina, even in cases where a person is so well-endowed that it reaches the cervix, the baby is still protected by the mucous plug, the length of the cervix and the amniotic sac.

So, while it may be a blow to the male ego, despite the length of a man' penis, it is not at all possible for an unborn baby to feel or be harmed by a penis during penetrative sex. Unless of course the cervix is dilated and the amniotic sac has ruptured (usually occurs during labor, in which case you should hold off on penetrative sex and concentrate on birthing!

Q. Fear of orgasming during birth?

EP: For some women the fear of birthgasms is real!

Orgasmic Birth or Ecstatic Birth are both terms coined to describe labor and birth that involve orgasms being experienced by the birthing person. I'm here to remind you how orgasms during labor and birth can help and why you should shake off the fear and embrace the "O Yes!".

Oxytocin is one of the hormones responsible for driving labor. It's sometimes referred to as the love hormone and is released during foreplay, sex and orgasms. During labor Oxytocin release peaks higher than at any other time in a woman's life, so it's no surprise that if we allow Oxytocin to flow freely orgasms might occur.

Now in theory this sounds great, but if you're in an unfamiliar environment, surrounded by near strangers, this scenario might sound a little bit intimidating.

Masturbation and orgasm during labor increase oxytocin levels, facilitating longer, stronger and more powerful uterine contractions. When the intensity of uterine contractions increase, so do our pain levels. One way to take the edge off is to elicit pleasure. Pleasure not only causes increased Oxytocin levels, it also encourages the release of endorphins, our bodies natural pain-relieving hormones.

The connection between birth and sexual pleasure are closer than you may have thought. So don't fear orgasm, embrace it.

Q. Fear of dying in birth?

EP: For some people the very thought of giving birth triggers such an overwhelming storm of emotions that they'll avoid pregnancy all together. This intense or severe fear of birth is called tokophobia. It's perpetuated by how we see labor and birth depicted in the media and It's not helped by friends and family, or the people around us that insist on telling us horror stories of their own experience of birth.

If you're feeling deathly afraid of birth there's a few things you can do to help you move past the fear.

1. Find an experienced care provider that you trust completely. Someone who respects your desires and fears and can confidently reassure you, and provide the care you need. If you don't have a deep trust in your care provider, reassurances will mean nothing.
2. Seek therapy before or during pregnancy. Talking to a trained professional about your fears and unpacking them can really help to alleviate the negative emotions you're holding onto.
3. Unsubscribe from the negative. It's totally ok to mute or unfollow social media accounts that might be adding to your anxiety and fears about birth. Avoid TV shows and movies that depict birth in a negative light and stop listening to podcasts that aren't serving you.
4. If friends or family want to share their birth story with you let them know "hey, I'd love to hear all about it, BUT if it's going to add to my fears or scare me, let's chat about it after my baby has arrived".

5. Educate yourself. Completing antenatal education can really help to expel some or all of the fears you might have. Knowledge gives you power. You might think that knowing the ins and outs and chatting through the 'what ifs' will just add to your fears, but for most people education helps them feel empowered and excited about what lies ahead.

Every person deserves to be excited about pregnancy and the birth of their baby. If you're feeling anxious and fearful of birth, I encourage you to do some, or all, of the above and try to get to a place of confidence and empowerment.

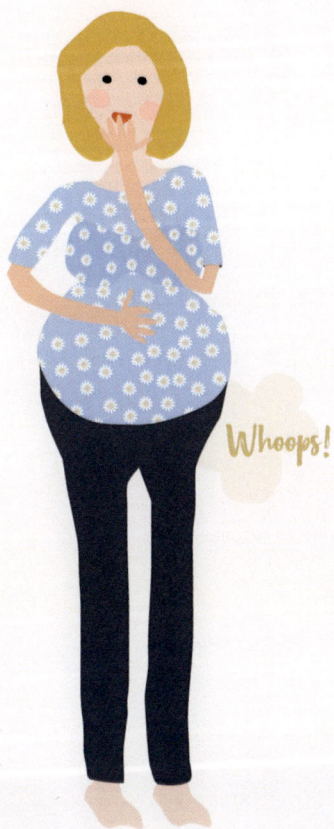

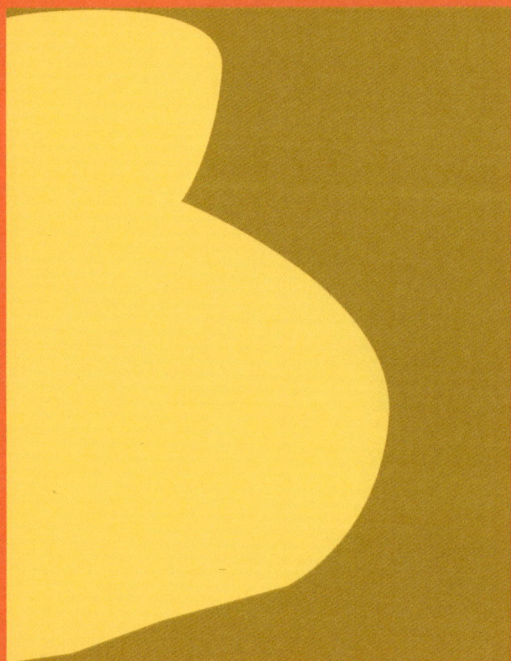

PLANNING FOR POSTPARTUM • PLANNING FOR POSTPARTUM

PLANNING FOR POSTPARTUM • PLANNING FOR POSTPARTUM

PLANNING FOR POSTPARTUM

PLANNING FOR POSTPARTUM • PLANNING FOR POSTPARTUM

PLANNING FOR POSTPARTUM • PLANNING FOR POSTPARTUM

'Mothers need support, so they then don't need to ask for help.'
– DR OSCAR SERRALLACH 2022

As I've now been down the postpartum road twice, and I've written a whole book on my personal thoughts about the postpartum experience (*AFTERWARDS*), I thought this book should cast a line out into the sea of 'What's To Come'.

I won't go into a huge amount of detail as that's what *AFTERWARDS* is there for, plus the many other fabulous resources on the market (books, poddys, blogs, web series such as The First Word etc), but I will touch on one of the most important aspects of the postpartum element. And that is, Planning for Postpartum. I have to admit I largely overlooked the need to plan for my two postpartum phases!

Isn't hindsight a wonderful thing? A bastard. But a wonderful bastard all the same.

Why plan & not just cross that bridge when you get there? Well, I guess you absolutely can since most of us do it that way (myself included)! Doing it that way however tends to bring a collection of unwelcome surprises … and let's face it. Everyone can benefit from a little foresight.

Sure, we all do it. We have babies and many of us go back and have more. During this procreating process however, what we don't do as well as we should, is recover … or allow adequate time & resources to recover well. And by that, I mean recover in ways that address both the *internal* and the *external* consequences of bringing babies into the world.

Believe it or not, eating 1 of the 20 lasagnes you'll be given after birth and watching back-to-back Netflix series, while dressed in an adult sized nappy with icepacks strapped to various parts of your body – is not 'recovering'. This is just plain old 'surviving'.

We women are so hard wired to get up & get on with it. Aren't we? We **always** put the baby and the entire family unit before ourselves, leaving our exhausted & frail bodies (and minds) to carry the weight of our selflessness. The issue here? Far too many of us become struck down with pre & postnatal depression, pre & postnatal anxiety, iron deficiencies, thyroid issues, hormonal imbalances, prolapse, incontinence or many other pelvic floor issues. Our automated response of just "getting on with it" can leave us utterly depleted, if we're not careful.

And depletion is no joke. I can speak to this with absolute experience.

When my second baby George was about 4 months old I started complaining of a kind of fatigue I'd never felt before. I was forgetting things (How to get to my toddler's daycare? Does shampoo or conditioner come first? Why did I come into this room? Where are my keys … Oh hang on, where is my car?). I felt completely dazed, despite finally getting some good sleep again. I looked pale, puffy and my eyes were heavy. I felt dizzy & discombobulated. I was a shell of a human. But there I was, like ALL other mums, just getting on with it. Because that's what you do when you're a mum.

People close to me suggested that perhaps I was simply adjusting to life with 2 children under 3? With time, my energy levels would regulate. Surely! And I thought the same. Until one Friday morning… I sat down and erupted in floods of tears in front of my husband & toddler. I felt embarrassed and nervous to say aloud, 'I am definitely not right. Something is wrong with me. It's as if I am going insane.'

Here I want to stop & quickly explain the embarrassment I felt in that moment, as I am sure SO many of you will relate to this either now, or when your baby is here… I have two healthy kids. A great marriage. A roof over my head and good friends. I am lucky to receive a lot of help from the grandparents and my toddler attends childcare two days a week. Despite this, I was STILL struggling?! Huh?

Some women have NO help! Some women live away from family! Some women are unable to afford childcare, or they don't have access to safe or dependable care during the day. Some women have kids with special needs who require parental care around the clock. And here I am with two healthy kids (who sleep), with loads of help and *I am the one to complain?! I'm tired?!*

What A Joke.

The tears fell. The shame filled the room. Luckily for me, I have a very supportive husband who reminded me that I was in fact not A Joke. I was someone who needed help. Not help with my kids – but help with my own health.

Needing help is a big thing for both a woman and a mother to admit, isn't it? We are not wired to lean on people. We are wired to allow people to lean on us. We are proud beings who Can Do It All. And there is truth in that. We CAN do it all. But even Superwoman needs a cape to help her fly.

To cut a long story short. I went to the GP, explained the way I was feeling and behaving (i.e. the way the memory loss was affecting my day-to-day i.e. putting the remote in the fridge, storing my dirty breakfast dishes under the sink… simply forgetting what I was doing up to 10 x per day).

I had my bloods checked and … oh my golly. Well, the problem was realised.

While my iron levels were 'ok' (very low but not dismal), my TSH (Thyroid Stimulating Hormone) levels were alarmingly off. My TSH levels should have been in the range of 0.4-4mU/L for someone my age (32). My levels were 155mU/L. Yes, 155. In short, this meant my thyroid was critically UNDERactive. I had my bloods redone to double check, as my GP was unsure the first tests could be right!

Sure enough, they were the same…Well actually, this time they were a little worse at 161mU/L. Three GP's *and* a Women's Health Naturopath said they had **never** seen such results. I've actually included an image of my results below. Why? To encourage everyone to ask that their health results are stored in their My Health Record account, accessible via MyGov.

Having access to your blood test results (and other health related results) is exceptionally powerful as it encourages you to **(A)** read them thoroughly & learn what it all means and; **(B)** get to know the inner workings of your own body.

Below, where you see RED, is where the lab has highlighted reason for alarm & where action needed to take place. You'll see a lot of RED in my case. Strangely I was not panicked by these alarming figures. I was relieved….."I'm not going crazy!!!! I am NOT going insane!" The sense of relief was remarkable. I had detected a problem and now I could focus on the fix.

Thyroid Function Tests

22nd Nov 2022

TEST NAME	RESULT	UNITS	REFERENCE INTERVAL
TSH	155 H	mU/L	0.4–4.0
Free T4	<5L	pmol/L	9–19

23rd Nov 2022

TEST NAME	RESULT	UNITS	REFERENCE INTERVAL
TSH	161 H	mU/L	0.4–4.0
Free T4	<5L	pmol/L	9–19
Thyroid Peroxidase Ab	285.8 H	IU/mL	<6
Thyroglobulin Ab	31.6 H	IU/mL	<4

So what did this all actually mean? My diagnosis was Severe Hypothyroidism, an auto immune disease which was possibly & probably triggered during my 2nd pregnancy, i.e. a period of time where my hormones were all out of whack.

The main symptoms of Hypothyroidism are set out below. I've noted my own experiences in italics.

* Tiredness. *Yes. On a whole new level. I wouldn't say I felt sleepy, but heavy. Lethargic. My bones felt dense & heavy. My brain felt slow and muddied. The collagen in my face felt (and looked) as if it had hit the snooze button.*
* More sensitivity to cold. *No, however keep in mind I was also breastfeeding which can affect your body temperature.*
* Constipation. *Yes.*
* Dry skin. *Yes, however again, keep in mind I was also breastfeeding which can contribute to dry skin.*
* Weight gain. *Yes. Despite being between 4-7months postpartum when I went through this experience, (and yes I do appreciate I'd very recently had a baby, a time when carrying additional weight is not uncommon), but I carried about 4-4.5kg more than usual. It wasn't 'baby weight' as I know where my baby weight sits ... there were just stubborn kilos that hugged my stomach & waist ... and did not budge.*
* Puffy face. *Yes. This was a huge tell tale sign for me. I kept saying to people 'my face ... it just looks different? I look like I've just woken up from a 20 hour sleep" ... and I did.*
* Hoarse voice. *No.*
* Coarse hair and skin. *Dry hair (although this is not uncommon for me).*
* Muscle weakness. *Yes. This was another tell tale sign for me. I cannot stress how hugely this symptom hit me. During a usual weights class I was completely unable to finish a 30 sec-1min session of weight lifting without stopping a few times ... I'm talking lifting weights as little as 1kg, or just my body weight(I.E. Lunge & squat sets). I've always been a fit & 'driven person' regarding exercise, so I could tell my body was not right.*
* Muscle aches, tenderness and stiffness. *Aches yes, stiffness no. Perhaps this was due to the presence of the relaxin hormone in my body as I was breastfeeding. Relaxin can soften your ligaments & joints.*
* Menstrual cycles that are heavier than usual or irregular. *N/A. I was breastfeeding & my period had yet to return.*
* Thinning hair. *Perhaps, but I grow a lion's mane so it was hard to tell.*
* Slowed heart rate, also called bradycardia. *Not in my case. In fact I went*

the opposite way thanks to my survival mechanism (albeit not a healthy one), OCD.

* Depression. *I felt 'down' and 'uncomfortable' because of what was happening, however coming from someone (me) who has had depression and who has been treated for depression, I knew very well that this was different. I could still feel joy & happiness. I wasn't numb. I was just ... utterly and completely exhausted & totally depleted.*

* Memory problems. *I can't stress how exhausting & concerning the memory loss was. Not to mention, alarming. I cried often, saying to my husband, 'I feel like I'm going crazy. I feel drunk... half the time I forget my own name.'*

... I have tears in my eyes as I write this, as this period of time was so hard. I had a beautiful family ... I was surrounded in great support ... I was finally getting sleep after losing almost 3 solid months of it thanks to baby George's Colic... and yet every single day, I felt loopy. I felt vague, dazed, confused, forgetful & a bit stupid to be honest. I lost a lot of confidence and self-esteem yet I didn't really speak to anyone about it because of **(A)** the shame ... ('Get on with it woman! You've got a great life and two healthy kids. You should be grateful. Now chin up and get going!" ... and **(B)** I didn't want to invite or perpetuate the advice and observations like...

* 'Well you do have a new baby & a busy toddler? Maybe you're just exhausted from this big life adjustment?'
* 'You've just resigned from your job of 10 years (which I did during this time), maybe the stress & fatigue from that big move is just hitting you now?'
* 'Maybe you have Postnatal Depression?'
* 'Maybe you're just struggling? Or you are not enjoying motherhood?'

The first 2 comments would irritate me as I know my body. And the more I heard comments of this nature (including a few from a male GP), the crazier I felt. Something was NOT right with me. I just wanted to scream from the rooftop, 'SOMEBODY, PLEASE LISTEN!'

The 3rd comment was a tough one to hear as well. I've dealt with depression since I was a teenager. I know my triggers as well as Bert knows Ernie. What I was experiencing was very different. How was I so sure? Despite the exhaustion I could still feel varied moods including joy. When depressed, joy is the first emotion to go.

The 4th comment would break my heart. What if people were right? Maybe I wasn't coping? What if I just wasn't cut out to be a mum of two.

Oh ... the latter gave me shivers.

Anyway, back to the mechanics of the diagnosis; Hypothyroidism.

Hypothyroidism is an auto-immune disease causing your thyroid to become underactive, or in my case, pretty much inactive. My GPs think I may have Postpartum Thyroiditis, which is a particular form of Hypothyroidism brought on by pregnancy. The good news is, is that this particular form of Hypothyroidism may resolve itself a few years.

First up, those of you who are unsure, your thyroid is part of your body's endocrine system, a system that is made up of glands that make hormones. The thyroid is the gland that controls your metabolism ... and your metabolism is the chemical process that breakdowns the food you consume to create energy. Your energy levels are then of course linked to your weight, your mood, your body temperature, your cycle, your sleep, your cholesterol, your digestion... your everything! In summary, when your thyroid is out of whack – your entire body is out of whack. And I can assure you, I was Out Of Whack!

Luckily for me and the many others who will cross paths with either Hyperthyroidism or Hypothyroidism in their lifetime, there is medication which is both very effective & readily available. So that is a HUGE plus! But dealing with a disease of this nature, with two small dependants in tow is comparable to holding a 10kg weight above your head for a very long time. Painfully uncomfortable.

My point?

Do yourself a very big favour & get to know the basic inner workings of your body before your baby is born. This way you'll be more aware if something is feeling 'off' during postpartum. Better yet? Ensure your partner learns this stuff with you! Post birth, the postpartum experience is theirs too. Your body carries your collective child. Therefore your body should be the collective responsibility of both parents. If you're a sole parent, lean on someone you know and trust to be your 'spotter' for like of a better term.

If I had my time again, during pregnancy I would have gone to the GP and asked for bloods to be taken to check the following at the beginning, middle & end ... just so I knew my 'base lines' and I could loosely monitor any drastic changes.

* TSH/T3/T4/Thyroid Antibodies/Thyroglobulin/Thyroid Peroxidase Ab
* Iron/Ferratin
* Haemoglobin
* Liver Function
* Lipids
* Glucose/C-Peptide
* Folic Acid

The following list covers what you could also check (via blood tests & in some cases urine tests), if your thyroid results sit outside of the 'normal' range. Listed below are the elements that support a healthy thyroid.

If you can get this stuff on track, your thyroid will be in a good position to keep working well. The goal!

* Iodine
* Zinc
* Vitamin B12
* Vitamin D
* Copper
* Magnesium
* Selenium
* Molybdenum
* Manganese
* Vitamin C
* Vitamin A
* Vitamin E and
* Vitamin K2

Again, if you understand your body, if you know your baselines, if you can detect deficiencies early and tend to these deficiencies throughout your pregnancy, come birth & life post birth, you'll be in a far better position to avoid depletion and *possibly* also postnatal depression. I emphasis the word *possibly* here as some things are out of our control. And best yet, you will simply FEEL BETTER. And what is better than feeling good?

The Cost Mentally
Huge.

Please remember that EVERYTHING to do with your physical self, can absolutely affect your mental self. The two go hand in hand. You'll hear about my personal collision of physical VS mental below*. Let me be an example of what can happen if you take your eye off the ball.

The Cost Financially
Huge.

Health is paramount, of course! In today's age however health care can also be very, very expensive – even with private health cover. This is even more of a reason to stress the importance of preventative measures, as we all know the best cure is prevention!

To give you an insight into how this diagnosis/depletion/postpartum experience cost me financially. The expenses included:

* 3 x GP appointments to find a GP who gave me adequate time & heard what I was saying i.e. a GP who didn't give me the TNM diagnosis i.e. 'Tired New Mum.' As GP appointments are charged based on time I was always paying for Long Appointments, which are not cheap.
* Another 2 x GP appointments once I'd found a great doctor who helped me get the necessary referrals for tests & further appointments.
* Clinipath Lab Tests (most tests are covered by Medicare but some are charged privately).
* Appointments with an Integrative Medical Doctor who specialises in Women's Health RE postpartum, thyroid & hormones issues. These

appointments were to monitor my bloods (taken every 6–8weeks) and manage my thyroid.

* Thyroxine Medication
* Supplements such as Iodine and Magnesium to correct what I was lacking (i.e. supplements that assist in the regulation of my thyroid).
* Therapy with a Clinical Psychologist* Now this one might not be relevant to everyone who suffers depletion or extreme issues with their hormones or their thyroid. In my case, babies aside, I've been treated for Depression & Anxiety for over a decade. My experience with anxiety in particular has always presented as OCD behaviour (Obsessive Compulsive Disorder). During the peak of my Hypothyroidism, my body went into fight or flight mode pretty much 24/7 … so despite the lethargy, I was getting hit with a lot of cortisol (the stress hormone produced by your adrenal gland). I became hyper manic, as my reliance on my OCD neuroses deepened, as this was my coping mechanism (…ordering things, repeating little mantras in my head, feeling as though I 'have to do something' to prevent 'something else bad happening' or to stop bad thoughts, touching something a particular number of times, making sure my arms or legs are crossed or uncrossed while doing particular things… it's a headache, trust me). My GP referred me to a therapist who could help using tools such as ERP therapy (Exposure Response Therapy) to combat the OCD while my body recovered from being quite unwell. This is great but therapy is expensive.

And don't forget;

* Childcare costs for carers to look after the tiddlees while I attended all of these medical appointments.

When you tally the cost of these appointments & medications … it's a hefty bill. Medicare does help via rebates & subsidised mental health appointments (x10 in Australia), but you're still out of pocket quite a lot.

TRANSITIONING TO 'MOTHER'

Here's a question for you. Are you familiar with the term, "matrescence"? I certainly was not, until I read a brilliant book called *The Postnatal Depletion Cure* by Dr Oscar Serrallach. The term 'matrescence' was coined by anthropologist Dana Raphael — and is defined as, 'the process of becoming a mother in terms of the physical, psychological, and emotional changes people go through during the monumental transformation that is motherhood.'

In other words, matrescence is the period of life when a woman becomes a mother. In short, just like adolescence – the period of time when a child becomes an adult, there is a huge surge of hormones that change & challenge us physically and mentally when we become a mother. Society focuses on and caters to adolescence , but somehow, matrescence, which is another difficult transition, is largely ignored.

Recently a friend said to me, 'when it comes to your health, you have to be your own biggest advocate'. So if society continues to ignore the matrescence period of life for women, you'll need to put your Big Girl Pants on, and speak up for yourself. If you know you are not right – seek help. You're not a tired, whinging mother nor are you a hypochondriac. You're a proactive mother, doing the best for your family.

My story isn't meant to scare you by the way! It's simply to alert you to the fact you may experience "additional" unplanned issues, when you become pregnant or during the postpartum phase.

On the following page is an extract from *The Postnatal Depletion Cure*, for added context and understanding.

WHAT IS POSTNATAL DEPLETION?

'Postnatal Depletion is a constellation of symptoms affecting all spheres of a mother's life after she gives birth. These symptoms arise from physiological issues, hormonal changes, and interruption of the circadian day/night rhythm of her sleep cycle, layered with psychological, mental and emotional components.' – DR OSCAR SERRALLACH 2022

Please be mindful when reading the below, that it is expected for women to feel a level of 'depletion' after the birth of their baby as they're tired, hormonal, sleep deprived ... the list goes on. In some cases however, (like my own), the feeling of 'depletion' will morph into something more sinister & beyond your control to manage alone, or with extra sleep/support. When and if you feel as if something is physically off, listen to your gut & visit your GP. Check your bloods and assess what's going on on a physical level. Don't ever assume, *'Oh I'm a mum now. This is just part of it.'* No, no, no. Trust your gut & prioritise your health.

Postnatal Depletion is not the same as being 'burnt out', or 'sleep deprived', or 'depressed.' The word Depletion originates from the Latin language and is defined by the "act of emptying or reducing.' In the postnatal context, Postnatal Depletion is a time of life where your body and mind are literally 'emptying' and 'reducing.' Every cell in your body is trying to recalibrate however due to the many (and I mean, MANY) changes to your body during pregnancy & birth, this process can lead to some serious complications. So please – do your best to prepare, plan and learn.

How to tell if you're suffering from Postnatal Depletion VS Postnatal Depression:

✳ If you are feeling exhausted, yet you're still able to 'feel joy' when moments in life bring goodness – this is likely Depletion. Those who suffer Depression will find their moods are very 'flat line'. Feeling joy and happiness will not be easy.

✳ Sleep is another good indication. If you are up during the night and able to fall back to sleep quite easily, this is likely Depletion. Those with Depression (despite utter exhaustion on a physical and mental level) will find it hard to silence the noise in their brain keeping them awake.

PLAN FOR POSTPARTUM

Below are a few of my ideas about how to plan for the postpartum experience ahead. These are only my personal suggestions, so don't forget to talk to the many mums you know for further hints. Based on their stories and experiences you will glean a world of wisdom!

✳ **Read *AFTERWARDS* by Tori Bowman Johnson** (Shameless plug? Guilty as charged!)

✳ **Visit your GP and ask for blood tests to check everything listed earlier in this chapter.** Detect any deficiencies early, and treat them to improve your health and your pregnancy, birth and postpartum experience.

✳ **Ask for your results to be uploaded on to your My Health Record** (via MyGov), so you have access to your own results. Visiting a GP, a naturopath, a physiologist, a physio … or anyone else in the medical/ wellness industry can be so much more value-adding when you can show them your actual (and most recent) results.

✳ **Line up your support network.** Sit and think … when and if the sh*t hits the fan, who are you going to feel comfortable calling on for help, or even just to talk to or vent with. We are all very good at soldiering on but if you let your frustration fester, you may find it will transition into rage.

✳ **Share the mental load!** Keep a list of what needs to be done around the house & make sure everyone contributes! If a visitor pops over and says 'How Can I Help?,' simply ask them to do something on the list. I'm sure unpacking the dishwasher OR folding some sheets is a very welcome contribution for most.

* **Assess the money you spend on household needs each week.** Is there a further investment the family could make to help you through a period of life where sleep is heavily reduced? A cleaner? ? Meal delivery services for a few weeks after the initial 2 weeks of bub's birth (I suggest 'after the initial 2 weeks' as you'll likely get a whole heap of beautiful people dropping off meals & snacks in the first few weeks).

  For those with other children, could you afford 1 extra day of childcare for the first 4-8 weeks of bub's arrival? If you don't have family around, is a Doula something you'd feel comfortable with?

  Can you invest in a REALLY comfortable nursing chair! A chair you'll genuinely crave sitting in as you feed all day and night? If you have anxiety around your baby's sleep, could it reduce your stress by booking a sleep trainer?

* **'You Time'.** Work out what this looks like for you personally. What makes you feel really relaxed? A walk? A facial? Brekkie alone at a cafe? A swim in the ocean? A long drive? Make a list of these things and make sure you fit in at least a few EVERY WEEK. One daily would be ideal but I'm a realist. Daily 'You Time' can be hard to factor in during the newborn days.

* **Try and find comfort in what I wrote above.** 'Daily 'You Time' can be hard to factor in during the newborn days.' Don't worry mummas! The newborn stage is not forever!! It's simply a phase of life that will change as bub grows.

As I've said so many times throughout this book, the subject of the chapter is not to make you fearful or angst ridden. My goal is the exact opposite. If you plan (and by this I mean plan loosely) for the postpartum journey, I promise you'll love yourself for doing so when you welcome your darling into your arms & into your home.

Think of it like a triathlon! The night before the big race you carb load, right? Postpartum planning is carb loading!! And who doesn't love a comforting bowl of good ol' spaghetti.

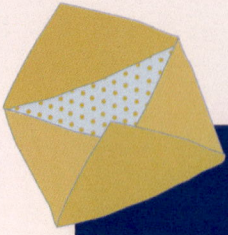

A Letter to Her Pregnant Self

FROM PHOEBE

This mother, Phoebe, is expecting her first child. While already a brilliant stepmother, she awaits a little person who will share her own DNA. Such magic ahead mumma, as you await the gaze of your adoring little.

While enduring the long days of pregnancy, a time when you feel heavier in the heart, mind & belly, Phoebe so gracefully sailed through. With a few unexpected hiccups rearing their testing heads along the way, with her strength & self assurance Phoebe writes herself a retrospective letter ... to offer the golden truth, 'it is all worth it'. Busy with flutters of cravings, hormones, kicks & turns, the journey of carrying her baby is one of delight.

Dear me,

Your pregnancy will be challenging, unpredictable, gratifying, and uniquely yours.

Weeks 1-19 of nausea but never sickness. The mind is a different story as you struggle to adjust to this new commitment. Know that it's okay to feel trapped, acknowledge the feelings that a last minute trip to Paris might not happen for you any time soon and throw them away. Because also, let's get real, when was the last time you took a last minute trip to Paris? The possibilities of living your 'old life' are now limited, but then, the possibilities of living a whole 'new life' are now endless. And sure, you wanted a daughter, but try to work on some perspective, you are lucky to be pregnant, that is all that matters. You have a stepson and you are growing a son, this is your life, it's good, and you will love it, love him, instantly, just you wait.

Weeks 20-24 of total shock, fear and disbelief as you learn that your cervix has shrunk from 38mm to 4mm. Cry, feel overwhelmed, breathe and take confidence in the skills of your doctors, who insert a tiny stitch that you all hope will hold your baby in place. Be grateful for your community, who rally around you as you're forced into bedrest until the baby is viable, and then beyond. Listen to your older, wiser sister and take comfort in her ever-practical advice that the 'whole point of being pregnant is to have a baby'. Because it's not about having a cute bump and enjoying this time, skipping around Melbourne. It's about surrendering to your circumstances, taking the pregnancy day by day, growing your child with the healthiest body and mind you can muster and balancing positivity with a considered dose of realism.

Weeks 25-34 of taking it easy, on yourself and your body. You're learning how to say 'no' to commitments, to important work, to a lot of fun, to things that it would have been easy to say 'yes' to a few months ago. Remember that this is training for the boundaries you will need to put in place in your fourth trimester.

Weeks 35-38 of racing through to-do lists, preparation and excitement. To breathing a sigh of relief that your baby is bigger, stronger now. You were so impatient for your pregnancy to be over, to get to full term. Understandable, as it wasn't an easy journey (whatever worth having is?). But you're here now, and you won't ever get this time again. This is it, your only experience of pregnancy and of birth. Slow it down and embrace this weird feeling. It will help to prepare for the uncertainty, stops, starts, highs and lows of motherhood.

In the end, you were right to worry, you were okay to be disappointed in your body initially and then overwhelmed by its strength and resilience in the end. You're actually going to make it through. And your body did exactly what you needed it to do, and then some. You'll understand soon enough what they mean when they say, 'it is all worth it'.

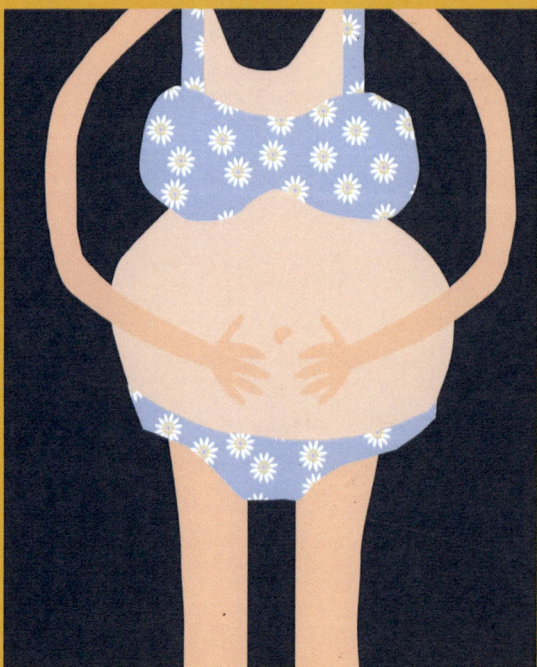

SIGNS OF LABOUR • SIGNS OF LABOUR

SIGNS OF LABOUR • SIGNS OF LABOUR

SIGNS OF LABOUR

The anticipation that coincides with the labor count down, is SO intense! While it's beyond exciting, it is utterly nerve-racking at the same time. As you wait to meet your baby for the first time the hours tick by so slowly. The mind races. The vacuum gets a solid workout as you go into an inevitable 'nesting mode' ... and the hospital bag creeps closer to the front door ... inch by inch.

Will it happen like in the movies? Will your waters break in aisle 7 of the supermarket? Will you begin showering your partner in colourful language if the contractions start to bust your balls? Will it hurt? Will it be fast? Will it be what you thought?

On this note, 'Will it be what you thought?' ... to be honest, it probably won't. This is not to say your labor story will be worse than expected. No way! But the thing about birth is ... no-one (not even your midwife or your OB) knows exactly how it will all pan out.

I did not expect to start my labor on all fours, first thing in the morning while trying to push my second born out. Ummm, god no!?! I thought I'd kick start comfortably, on my back wearing a cute sports bra or a fancy crop top that made my boobs look all perky & great. Yeah, that was not the case. I was on my hands and knees ... boobs hanging, hair flopping, sweat dripping, with the birth-end of the body spread for all to see.

It was primal, to put it delicately.

I had an audience (small, but an audience nonetheless) of cheerleader-like midwives watching on as if they were watching an episode of their favourite TV show. You have to love the midwives & their absolute love of birth don't you? I genuinely adore those women.

Anyway! I digress. If you do happen to have a birth plan that steps through your 'dream birth' second-by-second, rest assured even if the outcome deviates from your plan, your baby's birth will forever be special in the most wonderful of ways. Perhaps just keep an open mind should you need to alter your plan for a safe & healthy birth. The medical experts are experts for a reason.

Getting back to how will you know it's time?!

Thankfully the lovely Tahlia O'Rourke, founder of @wolfe.and.cub and our guest from Chapter 11 is back to share her knowledge!

Again, I'd like to preface that nothing below is to be taken as medical advice or direction. Anything & everything to do with your health, your pregnancy, your baby & your birth should always be checked by your personal GP, midwife or OB.

Q. Let's talk about the signs of labor! What are the most telling signs women should look out for?

Approaching full term, i.e. 37 weeks onwards, you may experience irregular 'period like' pain/cramping or lower back pain. Some women experience losing their mucous plug, diarrhoea, nausea or vomiting. Or of course some will experience their waters breaking. These can all be signs that labor is approaching.

Some mums express a feeling of just knowing something is different or something is coming. Whatever it is for you, follow your gut and go with it. Allow yourself and your body time to get into the rhythm of labor & rest when possible. Your body is about to run a marathon. Deep breaths.

Q. Braxton hicks can be tricky! Is there a way to decipher if they are BH or actual contractions?

Absolutely! Braxton Hicks are often referred to as "false labor." It's not uncommon for these types of contractions to send a mummy into the birth suite prior to being in active labor as it can feel similar to the real deal.

A Braxton Hicks is a tightening of the uterus, but with the absence of pain. You might feel your beautiful bump and think "gosh, that feels rock hard?!" ... but you shouldn't be experiencing any pain. Sure, they can be uncomfortable like any tight muscle, however by changing your position, having a warm bath or a shower, they should disappear. This is unlike contractions which will get closer together over time, stronger & there will be pain associated with the tightening.

Braxton Hicks do not cause the cervix to dilate. They're essentially a sign that your body is preparing for labor. What a wonderful & reassuring thing?!

Q. At what point should mumma call the midwife, her OB or her Doula?

Anytime your maternal instinct is telling you that something is not quite right, please pick up the phone. Waiting for your next appointment if you're having concerns, especially if your concerns are to do with your babies movements, is not wise.

You are your babies biggest advocate when they are womb-side (and let's face it, earthside as well!) so you must contact your lead care provider with any concerns.

Reasons to call the hospital include, but are not limited to:

* A decrease or a change in your baby's movements
* If you think your waters have broken
* If you experience bright red bleeding
* If you experience severe pain or feel generally unwell
* If you experience headaches, visual disturbances or extreme swelling
* If you experience strong & regular contractions that are painful. A good sign that you're in labor is if these contractions are five minutes apart & if they continue for at least one hour
* You feel ready to come to hospital. Never underestimate the power of what your gut is telling you.

Q. Is there ever a reason to rush just head to the hospital?

Yes. Severe abdominal pain, bright red bleeding, not feeling any movements from bub. If you experience any of these, just GO.

Q. Mums who are home alone & feel the need to drive themselves. Is this safe? Would a taxi or Uber be safer if they can't get hold of a loved one ?

If it is possible to have someone else drive you, this is the safest option. And that may even be an ambulance!

Side Note: You can always call an ambulance if you feel that your labor is progressing and you may be bringing your baby earthside in the car or on the side of the road. If this is the case, pull over, call an ambulance, put them on loudspeaker & follow their direction.

It's a good idea to always have a spare towel in the car just in case. Labor can be unpredictable at the best of times! Contractions experienced in active labor can take your breath away ... so driving is not recommended.

Q. **Can you explain the contraction aspect? When is it absolutely time to head to the hospital? i.e. how long between each contraction and how long will each contraction last?**

Contractions start off being irregular and short. This signifies early labor. They are all over the place at this stage ... they can be hours apart & last around 20-30 seconds each.

My personal 'golden rule' is that when you have been experiencing contractions that are strong, lasting 45-60 seconds each, painful & they recur like clockwork ...every 5 minutes, and they've been that way for at least 1 hour, then it's time to make your way to the hospital.

However, in saying that, every woman is different, everyone's perception of pain is different and everyone progresses through labor at different rates. If you feel ready to go to hospital and feel that will be your safe space, then call the hospital and head on in.

Some brave mammas might wait until contractions are 2-3 minutes apart & lasting 60-90 seconds each. It depends on how you feel and how you're coping.

There is no hard and fast rule.

Q. **While in labor at home, what can women do to stay calm & comfortable?**

Create an environment that is full of love and comfort and encourages your body to release the incredible hormone, oxytocin. The 'love' hormone.

Oxytocin is what makes the uterus contract, so if you can create a calm environment that supports the flow of that 'natural love hormone,' it can essentially help your labor progress & keep any adrenaline at bay. Adrenaline, during labor fights off all the beautiful work that oxytocin is doing. It can slow things down & prevent your labor progressing.

A few ideas to create a calming atmosphere include; dim the lights, light a candle (but don't forget to blow it out if you leave for the hospital ... LED candles or fairy lights are good for this reason), turn on a playlist of music you love. Practice deep breathing - in through your nose, out through your mouth! A relaxation massage is a nice idea, have a warm shower or a bath, utilise a heat pack, use a TENS machine or a fit ball. Use your bed for comfort (to lean into, to lean onto), and of course, rest when able. Diffusing essential oils like lavender, lemon or peppermint can be relaxing, uplifting & encourage contractions.

Have your support person present, encouraging you, affirming you, riding the waves with you and knowing when you want to make your way to the hospital.

Q. **For those at 40 weeks or over & wishing for their labor to start, can you recommend some initiation tactics? And is there anything they should avoid?**

Yep! I actually offer "The Wolfe Pack" on my website. The pack is a carefully curated birth kit that includes items to help mammas prepare and nourish their bodies for the labor and birth of their babies. It includes:

* Raspberry leaf tea and an infuser
* An essential oil roller with rose buds
* Pitted Medjool Dates
* A large gel heat pack with luxe linen cover
* Perineal ice packs
* A headband

Other ideas include:
* Go on a long walk (keep your phone with you in case you need to be collected!)
* Gutter walking (one foot on the gutter/curb, and one foot on the flat pavement).

* Gently bouncing on an exercise ball

The above are things to help your baby descend & engage in the pelvis.

The below ideas can help to boost Oxytocin. Remember, Oxytocin is the hormone that makes your uterus contract:
* Hand expressing
* Having sex

To soften the cervix:
* Eating dates
* Eating spicy food

To stimulate uterine activity:
* Drinking raspberry leaf tea

To tone the uterus:
* Acupuncture/acupressure

There are certain points that can help to induce labor:
* Organise a Membrane Sweep – aka a 'Stretch and Sweep' with your medical/birthing team

Some natural form of inductions for those interested:
* Anything that is going to heighten Oxytocin, again the love hormone. This could be to watch movies that evoke emotion, cuddling on the couch, surrounding yourself with your girlfriends and their babies or having a pregnancy massage.

This time is about you. This time is about nourishing you and preparing you to become a mother! Spend time with your partner, especially if this is your first, as you don't get that time back.

Try and avoid situations and/or conversations that place pressure on you or make you feel rushed to have your baby. That may mean asking your friends and family to kindly not message you all the time asking, "Have you had the baby yet?!" Kindly let them know that you prefer to tell them when your precious bundle arrives.

How you feel & how you are thinking in those final stages of your pregnancy is so important. It's a sacred time for you, your body, your baby & your birth partner.

Q. **When arriving at the hospital, what can women expect ? And should the partner drop mumma off at the front door before finding a park?**

It's a good idea to do a test run so you know how accessible parking is ahead of time, and where the best quick-drop area is. I am also a huge advocate for a tour of the birthing space before your due date. The reason being, if you are anything like me it is really reassuring to know where you are going to birth. A tour will also enable you to visualise the space before you're in labor awaiting the arrival of your baby.

Depending on how a mumma is feeling and progressing, having your partner drop you off VS walking in with you, is totally up to you. This really depends on the moment you arrive.

At most birthing facilities you'll be required to press a buzzer and wait for the door to be answered. Expect to be greeted by a member of admin or a midwife from the birth unit. Expect an initial assessment (we're pretty good at first impressions); then we'll place you wherever we feel best for your ongoing care. That might be in an assessment space or straight into a birthing suite!

Bring with you whatever you wish to have accessible during labor & birth.

Q. **Some women create a very specific birth plan, which is a lovely thing to do. However some women end up upset or disappointed if it doesn't go to plan. What is your advice around the birth plan?**

I'm a big advocate for women and their birthing partner writing down their birth wishes ahead of time, because often a birth won't follow the birth plan. If women make plans and fail to achieve them this can result in disappointment.

Birth wishes enable you to advocate for things you may wish to achieve when bringing your baby earthside. They can also make you feel educated & empowered

& give you the ability to advocate on your baby's behalf.

We can make wishes & hope they come true, whereas planning the birth can set up firm expectations.

Q. There are so many fabulous lists online regarding what to pack in the hospital bag. Is there anything a little left of centre that you'd personally recommend women bring into their labor?

Big black high waisted granny undies. That's it!

No in all seriousness, comfort is key. Bring along snacks – things that both you & your birthing partner love. This can provide a lot of comfort and 'feel good' emotions. Plus, sometimes you'll feel hungry for things other than hospital food.

Lip balm – hospitals are dry environments!

A personal idea from me (Tahlia), which some readers may like to adopt: The women in my life created a birth necklace for me. Each woman contributed a bead that they thought reminded them of me. We sat in a women's circle at my baby shower, opening the beads and talking about what they meant. It was so special to have something so unique to take with me to hospital, to encourage, inspire & motivate me. It now hangs proudly in my little boy's room.

Q. Emotions are high when labor starts, especially when pain & discomfort set in. It can be extremely distressing for the women ... who may revert to obscene language, anger towards the partner or a desire to just give up and go home. Of course, this is completely normal and OK! If a woman was to find herself distressed like this how can she calm down OR how can her partner help her to be calm?

It's a wild ride of emotions and hormones. As a midwife I always encourage a mum to stop, gain eye contact, engage, breathe and relax and know that each and every contraction is one step closer to meeting her beautiful baby. Sometimes a simple change of position or environment, suggesting getting in or out of the bath/ shower might be all she needs to shift and re-refocus her energy & emotion.

For partners, it can be extremely distressing seeing their loved one like this. Words of affirmation & encouragement, physical touch, offering refreshments and comfort, all help. Birthing partners should be a pillar of strength, for the woman in labor to lean on and lean into, so be that person.

Q. Lastly, if baby is showing signs of distress & an intervention is needed (for example forceps, the vacuum or a trip to theatre for an Emergency C section), is consent needed or must paperwork required be filled out etc?

Yes, absolutely. Like everything during your pregnancy, labor and birth, your birthing facility gain your consent constantly. It is your body & your baby. Verbal & written consent are a part of preparing for any procedure. In the case of a caesarean, written consent is required and you will need to sign a theatre consent form.

The Life Admin Check List

This list is in no particular order ...

- ☐ If applicable, have you enquired or registered for Paid Parental Leave from the government or looked into other government funded subsidy options?
- ☐ Have you done everything you want to do FOR YOU?
- ☐ Hair Appointment
- ☐ Waxing / Laser
- ☐ Mani / Pedi? Personally I wouldn't worry about this, as you probably won't have the time to get the colour removed or fixed for at least 3-4weeks post baby
- ☐ Walked around aimlessly?
- ☐ Have you downloaded some movies or TV series for the hospital in case they don't have wifi (which they likely won't)?
- ☐ Have you purchased & stored a tin of formula just in case you need it? Note here, you'll also need a bottle (might sound obvious, but nothing is obvious when you're busy growing a baby). Warning: Don't open the formula tin until you need it as formula has a very short shelf life after the seal is broken. It's helpful to write both the date you opened it & the date it will expire on the can to prevent any accidents.
- ☐ Have you checked that your Medicare and private health insurance information (if relevant), is all up to date? Remember that when baby is born, you'll need to add them to your Medicare, so it's best to get this stuff organised now ... and perhaps even set up a MyGov account if you don't currently have one & if you're in Australia. When baby is 6 weeks and you head to the GP for the 6 week check up (for both mum & bub), make sure to take your new Medicare card. If you don't have the new one by that stage let the GP know & keep all of

the receipts so you can claim the available rebates as soon as it comes in.

☐ Have you or your partner worked out the safest & most efficient route to the hospital? Avoid roads with multiple speed bumps or traffic lights. When you're in labor and experiencing contractions, these hold ups will feel as if the world is trying to prank you. And have your timed how long the journey is?

☐ Is your hospital bag packed? Have you worked out what the hospital does NOT supply for women? For example it's a good idea to check if they provide maternity pads, masks (for COVID reasons), a bath towel, a pool (should you be planning & preparing for a water birth), soap, toothpaste, particular types of tea & snacks.

☐ Have you reminded your partner where the vacuum lives & how to turn it on & use it? Do they know where the washing line is? Do they know that any existing toddlers or kids in the house require meals, snacks, baths & many changes of clothes every single day?

☐ Have you created a Breastfeeding Box should you wish to breastfeed? Find this must-have list in AFTERWARDS ... but in short it's a little box you create with everything you might need whilst you feed.

☐ Think about the postpartum ride ahead & perhaps familiarise yourself with the Planning For Postpartum chapter. Another shameless plug, but reading AFTERWARDS is a good way to plan!

☐ Have you asked your friends for a list of great podcasts to listen to during those late night/early morning feeds? Note Here; Perhaps stick to content that is on the lighter side. Murder mysteries can wait.

☐ Have you safely installed the baby car seat & had it checked by a professional? This is a requirement for some hospitals so make sure this is done around the week 32–35 just in case!

- [ ] Have you booked a Baby First Aid Course? If not, PLEASE DO!
- [ ] Have you purchased an extra long phone charger or a portable charger so you can remain connected & charged at all times (if you wish too of course!)
- [ ] Have you popped some frozen meals in the freezer (or asked a love one to do this for you?) Curries, lasagnas, risottos, bread, boobie cookies, pastas ... think of comfort foods!
- [ ] Have you read at least one positive birth story that made you feel all warm & clucky inside? DO IT! Read 100 if you can ... there are SOOOO many out there! Despite what society loves to tell us, birth is phenomenal!!
- [ ] Following on from the above point, have you realised that the best day in your life is about to come? And I mean, the VERY BEST?
- [ ] Ok, now do yourself a favour. Get up & go to your bathroom to check your stock levels. If you're like me and you buy a particular shampoo & conditioner from a salon rather than a supermarket or pharmacy, check that you have enough to last a few weeks or months. Maybe just buy a new bottle of each so you know you won't run out. Same goes with your face cleanser, moisturiser, serums, masks and lip balm. Sure, you can buy it all after the birth, however knowing that you're well stocked up is calming (well, for me at least). I bought about 10 pots of Carmex lip balm and put one in every single room of the house. I also put a pot in all bags, the car, the pram. Everywhere! Same goes with maternity pads. Anything you know you'll be using daily – stock up!
- [ ] Now, please exit the bathroom & head into the laundry and kitchen & check the cupboards. Do you have enough washing powder, toilet paper? Spray and wipe, dishwashing liquid, paper towels? Again ... yes you can buy all of these things after the

birth, but if I've learned anything after two babies, it's that going to the shops in the first month isn't easy. And going to the shops for these types of mundane things feels like such a waste of a rare outing. Save your trips out for coffee dates & walks in the fresh air.

☐ Now, let's head into your wardrobe. Do you have enough comfortable clothes to see you through? T's, supportive bike shorts, a robe (for feeding & quick coverups if and when people pop in & you're topless), warm trackies, thick socks? You don't have to break the bank with these items by the way … and to be honest I wouldn't. Beautiful lounge wear is very 'in Vogue' … we all know that (thanks COVID!), but don't waste your pennies on labels in this space as everything will be splashed with milk, food, sweat and snot in the very near future. Everything cops a thrashing in the machine & wears very quickly … so buy smart.

☐ Last but not least, have you practiced the phrase 'Yes Please?' When the baby arrives & people rush to help, whatever they offer to do or to bring you, just say 'Yes Please!' Try not to waste any energy fighting it. I didn't learn this until baby number 2, and let me say … saying, 'Yes Please' is a blessing!

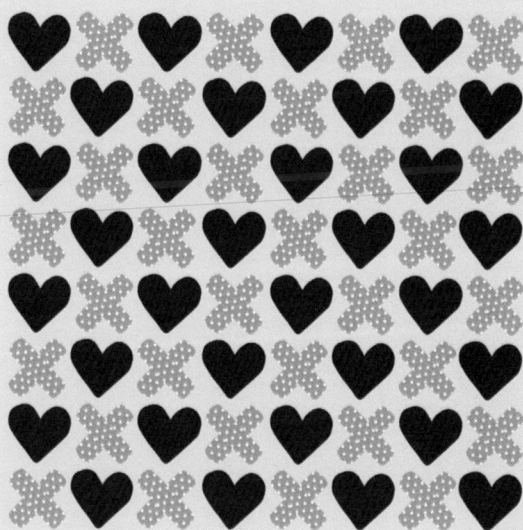

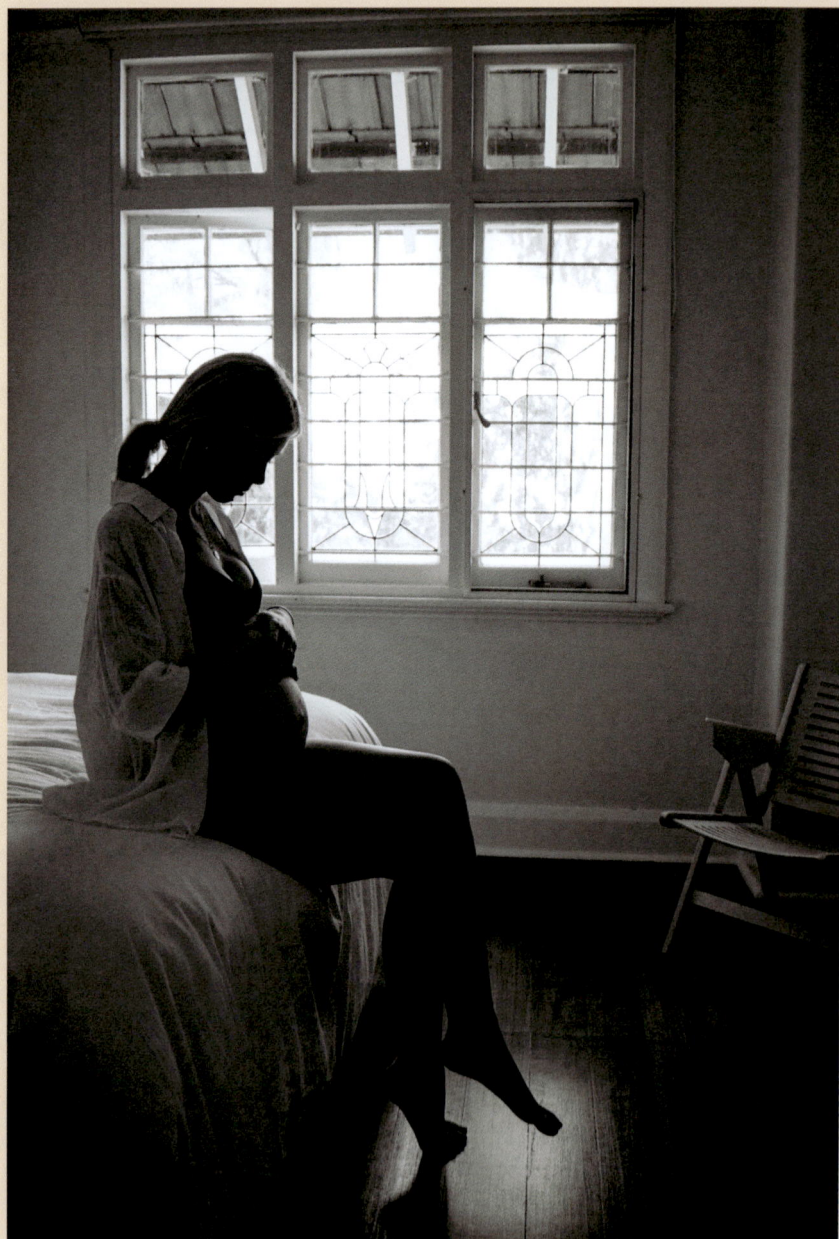

THANK YOU'S

Thank you to everyone who has shared their time & expertise within the pages of this book. The words of *BEFORE* started to spill out onto pages when I was just 7 weeks pregnant with my second baby, and they continued to spill onto the pages 9 months into my postpartum experience. Through the sleepless days & nights, carrying puffy eyes & a very discombobulated inner compass ... the goal of getting this book into the hands of those going through the ups & downs of fertility, pregnancy, birth and postpartum experience ... was never shadowed by the fatigue I felt. Connecting with women through writing has become a priority, because it is such a privilege to do so.

To all of the incredible professionals who have been credited in each chapter, your dedication & love of women's health, women's comfort & their overall happiness is nothing short of inspiring. From myself & on behalf of everyone who reads this book, thank you so much. I'm in utter awe of your skills & knowledge.

To my wonderful illustrator, Catherine. You have always nurtured such a gorgeous & creative talent, which I obviously adore. To say that you make the pages of both *BEFORE* and *AFTERWARDS* come to life, is an understatement! You have peppered my words with sensational sprinkles of colour. Each and every one of your illustrations is sweet yet wholesome, oh so delicious. Thank you. I can't wait to see what we do next!

To my designer, Jacqui at Northwood Green. You are so chic, so sophisticated, so on point. Your eye for colour, detail & unique design ... your graceful workstyle & your immaculate efficiency are all traits I very much look up to. As a working mother yourself, you showcase no limit. Thank you for joining me on this adventure & re-living the bump & baby days! I feel very grateful to have worked with you.

To my editor. My MUM (hi Mum as you're probably spell checking this!)! Yes, my very own mum edited my book. The same woman who taught me to read & write all those years ago. Mum is the ying to my yang and quite simply, my biggest fan and the feeling is mutual. Thank you mum for reading chapters written about sex! Thank you for reading through my mental health hiccups, which I am sure must be difficult on some level. Thank you for taking such amazing care of my boys and allowing me the time & space to write these books. And, thank you for showing me how to be a great mum. A fierce protector. A moral compass. A good person. You're a gift mum. My gift.

To my husband. Will, without you I would have nothing to write about! For giving me the opportunity to become a mother & to welcome such darling children into our lives ... oh my golly, I couldn't be more grateful if I tried. Babies aside, you are my home-sweet-home Will. You encourage me to explore, to *'just give it a crack'* & to dig deep into my never ending curiosities. You never doubt me. Not ever. I love you to infinity, and I simply adore our life together.

To my family, friends, medical team (my midwives, GP's etc), working colleagues, and every single individual who has ever helped me become & be a mother ... where would I be without you all!!! Without my wonderfully wide & warm village ... I'd be a mess. Such love is shared with all of you.

To my boys. My little dudes, Hamish Spencer (3y) and George James (9m).

I love you both to the moon and beyond ... or as Hamish says, "I love you big, so much."

Hamish. Where to start kiddo?! Your curious, assertive yet divinely sweet nature makes my heart do the waltz. You make me laugh – oh dear god, do you ever!! You make me wonder, imagine & question. You make me stop & smell the roses. You make me so proud. Please keep making everyone your friend. Ask them their names & their favourite colour ... and like you always do so eloquently, follow up with, *'It's nice to meet you!'* Share your 'cuggles' with everyone & never let the world tell you 'no'. Whatever you want to do in life kiddo, do it and do with pride.

George. You are glorious joy, wrapped in warm & fuzzies. You are quite simply the happiest baby the world has ever seen & you remind us of this daily. You are SO generous with your smiles and you are SO brave on those chubby little legs of yours. You are a go-getter. You're determined, you're strong and you are infinitely infectious. Your patience is mesmerizing. Your resilience is pure. Your calm demeanor has become my absolute peaceful haven. George you sweet thing, you're fabulous. Thank you for joining our family.

And finally, to every single woman reading this book ... you are, or you will become such a specular mother. Keep following your gut, keep showing yourself kindness and keep making the time for things that make you happy & that make you, you. Pour that wine at 4.59pm and know that I am always cheers'ing with you! Thank you for sharing your precious time with me.

For now, adios amigos! Maybe there will be a third book, maybe there won't! We'll just have to wait & see won't we!

With love,

Tori x

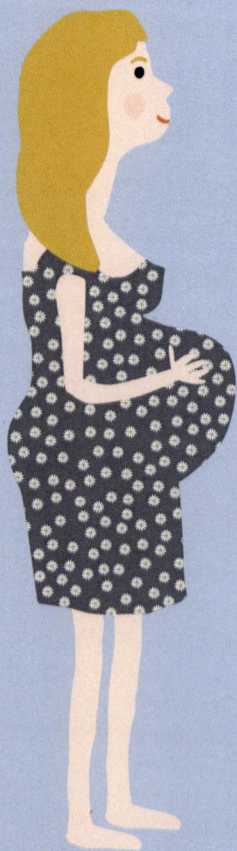

'There is no need to rush.
What is meant for you,
always arrives on time.'
— UNKNOWN